YOGA
FOR
WOMEN

YOGA FOR WOMEN

WELLNESS AND VITALITY AT EVERY STAGE OF LIFE

SHAKTA KHALSA

PHOTOGRAPHY BY RUSSELL SADUR

CONTENTS

A NOTE FROM THE AUTHOR

I adore teaching women yoga. Yoga and women go together like tea and toast. It's a cozy, homey fit. Women love to relax with other women. We love to share our experiences with each other, and after a yoga class, there are often much inspired and somewhat intimate conversations around. Someone is sure to say, "Wow, I needed that class!"

Just on the other side of yoga's relaxing coziness is its dynamic, transformational power. During the many years that I've been practicing yoga, I have grown in ways that I never would have imagined possible. I am not the same person I was—literally. I believe the atoms and molecules in my body are different than they were before I began a life of daily yoga practice. Life is so much easier, not because it doesn't present challenges, but because I can handle the challenges now. My ability to move on from life's crises I attribute to the consistent, honest work—and joy—of a daily yoga practice.

The key word is "daily." Don't let this intimidate you. Start out by thinking of it as a "steady" practice, 10 or 15 minutes a day, an hour every few days or so. You may experience a new and positive outlook that becomes more permanent. Emotions even out. Little things, and even big things, no longer hold the same power over you that they used to.

Such is the healing and transformational power of the yoga that is held within these pages. And now, if you are ready, let's begin.

Shakta Khalsa

Shakta Khalsa

Medical conditions

Practice yoga gently and slowly and include the use of recommended props—or avoid certain poses altogether—if you have one of the following medical conditions.

• Heart conditions and asthma: Avoid breathing exercises and aerobic or strenuous poses.

• Spinal conditions and osteoporosis: Avoid strenuous backbends, inverted poses, spinal twists, and balancing poses.

• High-risk pregnancy and postpartum complications: Check with your physician before starting yoga.

• Balancing problems and neurological diseases: Avoid poses that require balancing, especially on one foot or on the hands.

Remember, yoga is noncompetitive, so practice only to your capacity. Some restrictions may apply, depending on your physical abilities. If a pose causes discomfort, stop and go on to another pose, or do the easy-does-it version if one is provided. Always consult your physician with concerns you may have about any poses or exercises before doing them.

INTRODUCING WOMEN'S YOGA

Within the pages of this book, you will find a practical manual for nurturing the many facets of you as a woman. Yoga, as you may know, is an ancient art and science that brings health and well-being to your body, mind, and spirit. Yoga accomplishes this through a practice of movements, held postures, breathing exercises, and mental focus. People who practice yoga say that they feel more relaxed, accomplish more with less stress, and feel in touch with their inner being—their sense of authentic self.

WHY YOGA FOR WOMEN?

Yoga is good for everyone—men, women, and children. Why, then, a yoga book just for women? We women have well-defined needs, issues, and stages of life. Just think for a moment about how a woman's outlook and physical health are affected by her hormones, which control menstrual cycle, pregnancy, and menopause. Yoga balances these hormones efficiently and effectively through the stages of a woman's life. But yoga is not just for the bodily changes that women undergo. It is for balancing emotions and for the feminine need to have a cozy, relaxed way of life supported by a spiritual outlook. It has also been shown to be a gentle and consistent support for women's health. In this book, we will use yoga to address conditions that often affect women—depression, osteoporosis, arthritis, menopausal symptoms, heart disease, premenstrual symptoms, breast health, and memory loss, among others.

About 72 percent of those who practice yoga are women, and we are attracted to it for many reasons—to find relaxation, gain energy, and remain flexible physically and mentally, nurturing the spirit and developing inner strength and higher awareness. Generally, women exhibit more physical and mental flexibility than men. To be able to carry and birth babies, we have been designed with flexible bodies. We have an innate capacity to do many things at once—take care of a sick child, cook, talk on the phone, and perhaps three other things all at the same time. We have a natural mental flexibility that allows us to "go with the flow." These star qualities shine brightly with a practice of yoga and meditation that can be enhanced by beautiful, inspiring music designed especially for use with this book (see Music Resources, p.224). And through yoga, we experience the balanced interplay of vitality and relaxation—the ability to be alert yet peaceful, relaxed and energized, all at the same time.

As women, we also have needs. I have found from my years of practice and teaching that yoga goes directly to the heart of women's needs. We need to feel loved. Yoga develops self-love. We need to feel secure. Yoga lets a woman know her security lies within. We need to feel fulfilled. Yoga develops self-awareness and self-fulfillment. When a woman knows she is complete in herself, all of her relationships enjoy the benefit of that knowledge. Just with her presence, she uplifts her partner, her children, her parents, her coworkers, her friends, and even those she meets in passing.

I believe that you will find *Yoga for Women* to be a treasure trove filled with the best gems and jewels that women's yoga has to offer.

Remedies & more

In this book, you will find healing remedies and recipes based on the ancient science of yoga. These include:

• A tasty recipe for golden milk made with turmeric, an Indian spice that is known to keep joints lubricated.

• Special drinks for a woman in the first few days after giving birth, which will give her energy, will be easy on the sensitive digestive system, and will optimize the nutritional content of her breast milk, providing the richest nourishment for her new baby.

• An ancient recipe for a wonderfully luxurious yogurt bath that cleans your skin down to the pores and keeps you feeling and looking both young and relaxed.

• A soothing and delicious recipe for date milk to help wean babies, give energy, and help ward off colds.

BEGINNINGS

The genius of yoga is that it is a
self-perpetuating system. I have found that in
practicing yoga, I feel inspired and empowered to
want to do more yoga. It is as if yoga says to me,

"You take the first step, and let me do the rest."

Of course, experience is everything. So set yourself
up in a quiet space and get ready to begin your
yoga journey.

Here, at the beginning, is always a good place
to start. In this part of the book, you will come to
understand the big picture of yoga and begin to
glean many of the finer points that make yoga the
wonderful, self-transforming practice that it is.

THE BASICS

Yoga is older than recorded time. It may well be tens of thousands of years old. Yoga's beauty lies in the realization that a practice of yoga is as relevant to our lives in the 21st century as it was all those many centuries ago—maybe even more so, given the stresses and uncertainties of our fast-paced, modern lives. If I were to name one thing that has been the greatest blessing in my life, I would say it is my daily yoga practice and meditation. I like to practice in the quiet early morning hours, finishing up just as the light creeps across the sky and the birds begin their morning call. Throughout the day, when things are challenging, I sometimes recall how I felt early that morning and recapture that peaceful clarity.

The practice of yoga is so well known that it hardly needs explanation. But what, in essence, does yoga mean? Being an inquisitive sort of person, I always enjoy delving into the origin of a word in order to glimpse its essential meaning. The word "yoga" comes from the Sanskrit word *yug*, which means "to yoke," or bind together. And what does yoga bind together? All the various parts of ourselves, often thought of as body, mind, and spirit. Yoga is an instrument of wholeness. And by the way, did you know that the word "whole" is the origin of the words health, heal, and holy? Amazing, isn't it, how even an ordinary dictionary can be a source of enlightenment.

The main focus of this book is instructional, working with asanas (postures and exercises), pranayama (breathing techniques), and the practice of meditation. These are the tools of yoga—tools to pick up and use to change ourselves for the better, to let go of self-defeating patterns, and to live to our deepest and highest idea of who we are. As you move deeper into your practice, still more elements of yoga come in to play (see Yoga sutras, right).

UNDERSTANDING HATHA AND KUNDALINI YOGA

Although kundalini yoga has been the primary style of yoga I've practiced and taught for many years, I also very much enjoy my practice of hatha yoga. My vision in shaping this book is to create an artful, harmonious blend of hatha and kundalini yoga. The idea is to take the best of both worlds, although in reality hatha and kundalini are both from the same world of yoga, using many of the same postures and following the same yogic teachings. But for those of you who may be new to yoga in general, or to hatha and kundalini yoga specifically, I have included some background and basics about each yoga style here.

Yoga sutras

The science of yoga was known and practiced but not clearly documented until around 200 CE, when a physician-sage called Patanjali systematized and codified the science of yoga into what became known as the yoga sutras:

• **Yama** encourages moderation and restraint.

• **Niyama** gives the ground rules for self-discipline and inner awareness.

• **Asanas,** or yoga postures, keep the body healthy and the mind calm, creating an atmosphere in which the life energy can flow more easily.

• **Pranayama** focuses on experiencing the link between the breath, mind, and body.

• **Pratyahara** is the process of becoming aware of, and learning to control, thought patterns.

• **Dharana** is when the mind, once withdrawn into itself, is fixed in one-pointed inner concentration.

• **Dhyana** is meditation without focus on an object, founded in a deep inner space of awareness.

• **Samadhi** is the ecstatic state of being in which the meditator becomes one with the object of meditation.

Different yoga styles

The plethora of different styles of yoga is enough to make your head spin. Try to think of them as rays of light emanating from the same sun, and because they are from the same source, they are all related. It is only natural, though, that distinct differences between the various schools of yoga have developed over time, and thankfully so—there's something for everyone when it comes to yoga.

Unseen energy centers

According to the science of yoga, the body is made up of centers of energy called chakras that are not visible to most of us. Those who can see chakras say that these fields of energy are like fluid whirlpools of light, each with its own color, which are constantly moving and changing in complex patterns. Chakras function as intake organs for energy from the universal life force (prana) that is all around us. There are eight chakras (see sidebar, opposite).

ABOUT HATHA YOGA

The word "hatha" comes from two Sanskrit words, *ha*, meaning sun, and *tha*, meaning moon. Hatha yoga blends the sun/male/active energy with the moon/female/receptive energy that is in each of us.

Hatha yoga practice consists of held and moving postures, called asanas. There are a wide variety of asanas (over 200), each one with its own distinct form dictated by stretching, counterstretching, and resistance. The alignment of the muscular and skeletal structures is a major focus of the asanas. Adding a conscious breathing pattern to the postures helps circulate energy and blood and brings balance to the sympathetic and parasympathetic nervous systems, which govern the function of just about every other system in the body. In other words, asana practice is the key to the body, which is the key to the mind, which is the key to the spirit.

There are a wide variety of hatha yoga styles and traditions. Most of the hatha yoga included in this book is general, with some influence from the viniyoga tradition. *Vini* can be translated from its original Sanskrit word to mean individual. It can also mean step-by-step and gradual. With viniyoga, the pace is relaxed and poses are adjusted to meet individual needs.

ABOUT KUNDALINI YOGA

Kundalini comes from the word *kundal*, which means "lock of hair from the beloved." The uncoiling of this "hair" is the awakening of the kundalini, the creative potential that already exists in every human. The easiest way to understand kundalini is to realize that there is the universal spirit, sometimes referred to as God, that uncoils him/her/itself. This uncoiling process is known as kundalini. What is uncoiling and awakening is you, nothing more and nothing less. It is an innate capacity that most people simply are not utilizing. Yoga is the science of the self, and kundalini is the awakening of the self. It is that simple.

Poses that turn the body upside down, such as the shoulderstand, are called inversion asanas. Inversions are beneficial for boosting circulation and helping the lymphatic system to drain.

Chakras

- **The first chakra** at the base of the spine is our "root," grounding us on the earth, and relates to primal needs.

- **The second chakra** is located beside the reproductive organs and relates to sexual energy and creativity.

- **The third chakra** is at the navel and relates to stamina, willpower, and well-being.

- **The fourth chakra** is at the center of the chest, the heart center, and relates to personal and universal feelings of love.

- **The fifth chakra** is at the throat and relates to the ability to speak truth.

- **The sixth chakra** is at the center of the forehead where the eyebrows meet, known as the "brow point," and relates to the power of intuition and visionary qualities.

- **The seventh chakra** is located at the top of the head at the crown and relates to the all-expansive merger with the universal spirit.

- **The eighth chakra** is sometimes considered to be the aura, or electromagnetic energy field surrounding the entire body, as well as interpenetrating each of the seven other chakras in the body.

Tips for your yoga practice

- It is best to practice yoga barefoot on a nonslip mat with a blanket or rug for extra padding.

- Warm up with exercises in Warming up to Yoga (pp.30–41) before practicing a yoga set.

- Let your eyes focus softly or be closed. Turn your attention inward.

- Move slowly into the pose to avoid injury and to increase your inner awareness. If the instructions are to move quickly, build up to a fast pace as much as you are able.

- Discomfort is okay; pain is not. Stretch as far as is comfortable. Work on the edge of the stretch, but back off if you experience pain.

- Breathe, breathe, breathe! Unless instructed otherwise, inhale and exhale through the nose, not the mouth.

- Hold the poses for the minimum time if you are new to yoga, eventually working up to the maximum time.

- To conclude an exercise or posture, inhale and pause the breath briefly, then exhale and relax the posture.

The main aim of hatha yoga is to bring about a balanced flow of energy through the body's energy centers, called chakras (see sidebar, right). But, besides the energy that is already flowing within our bodies, there is a vast reservoir of untapped energy stored (according to yogic tradition) under the fourth vertebra of the spinal column. This latent energy is activated through kundalini yoga.

This untapped energy is stimulated through the proper practice of kundalini yoga as given by my teacher, Yogi Bhajan. As you maintain a steady yoga practice over a period of time, the energy gradually rises up the central column of the spine, balancing the body's chakras and activating the secretion of the pineal gland, which is located in the center of the skull. Although the pineal gland has remained an enigma in Western medicine, in yogic science it is considered the very key to life, both physical and spiritual.

Kundalini yoga, which includes many of the same postures found in hatha yoga, provides a good challenge yet is very doable; the positive effects can be experienced in a matter of minutes. It consists of both held postures and active exercises, often coordinated with strong breathing patterns.

MENTAL FOCUS DURING YOGA

During yoga practice, hold your mind in the present moment by keeping your attention focused on each breath that you take: you can hear it, feel it, even visualize the breath. As you inhale, see prana—or life energy—entering your body and mind. See and feel it as sparkling light, vital and fresh, bringing all possibilities to you. As you exhale, release the apana, the used-up energy, old thoughts and feelings, tensions, discomfort, and anything you are ready to let go of to make way for new beginnings on the next inhale.

As well as listening, feeling, and visualizing your breath moving in and out, you can also imagine hearing a sound on your breath. One sound that is often used in yoga is *Om*. Another is *Sat Nam* (rhymes with "but mom"). *Sat* is heard on the inhalation, and *Nam* on the exhalation. This means

"Truth is my/our essence." You can practice using affirmations in your own language that speak to you— for example, "I am, I am."

RELAXATION AND MEDITATION

Following the natural flow of a yoga routine, a period of deep relaxation and then meditation balances energy perfectly in the body and mind. A meditative mind and a relaxed mind go together: your relaxation practice will enhance your meditation, and the practice of meditation will teach you to relax. The yogic teachings say that there are different "processing" times needed to create certain desired effects during meditation. Although some meditations are given for a specific amount of time and should not exceed that time, most meditations are done for 11 minutes, which adjusts your pituitary, or master gland, and your nervous system, and also changes your outlook for the better. After 31 minutes of meditation, your entire mind and all the chakras are positively affected. After a 62-minute meditation, your subconscious mind is positively transformed and integrated with your conscious mind.

Each chapter in this book is designed as a beautiful and effective dance of yoga and meditation, set to the tune of women's themes. As much as possible, leave time at the end of your practice for at least 5 minutes of meditation, and preferably 11 minutes.

Starting your day with yoga can make a very real difference to how well your day goes. Some women find an afternoon practice rejuvenates and relaxes them for the rest of the day. Many women, especially those with children, find that their favorite time to turn to yoga is in the evening when the house is quiet. However you can squeeze your yoga time into your busy life, I guarantee that the effort will be worth it.

Relaxing with yoga

• Twenty seconds to a minute of relaxation between postures allows the energy to circulate throughout your body and mind.

• Follow your practice with a deep relaxation on your back for a minimum of 10 minutes, or more if possible.

• The optimal time for meditation is after your yoga practice, usually after a period of relaxation.

• Above all, enjoy. A little smiling goes a long way!

Yogic cycles of time

The yogic teachings talk of specific cycles of time that help change old habits and develop new ones. For a really special experience, you can choose a specific yoga set or meditation in this book and commit to a program of practice for one of the following times:

• **40 days** will change an old habit into a more positive one.

• **90 days** confirms the new habit in you.

• **120 days** allows the habit to become who you are.

• **1,000 days** ensures that you have mastered the habit.

BASIC POSTURES

Knowing how to sit is a very important component in yoga and meditation. Your sitting posture should provide a firm base for your spine to stack up straight. Why is this important? Think of a garden hose. When it is straight, the water flow is strong; when it is curved or twisted, the water flow is weak. In a similar way, your spine conducts spinal fluid, which nourishes every nerve and carries messages to your brain. Spinal fluid also contains prana, the Sanskrit word for the life force energy that flows through all of your body's energy centers, enlivening your vital awareness and your sense of self.

Straightening your spine is a matter of paying attention to how well your vertebrae are lining up. You can help this process by slightly tightening your abdominal muscles to hold the pelvis in place while lifting your breastbone slightly, and subtly pulling your chin in toward your neck to straighten the cervical vertebrae. Keep your shoulders relaxed. Visualize your spine lengthening and straightening, and relax into the feeling.

YOUR YOGA SPACE

Think of your yoga space as your personal sanctuary—a place where you can drop everything and be in a haven of peace. You may like to decorate a low table or altar with objects such as a candle, meaningful photos or objects, and a vase of flowers. If you don't have a particular place set up for yoga, just find a quiet spot where you will have room to move. Spread out a mat that will fit the length of your body, perhaps adding a blanket for padding. If you have a hardwood floor, use a nonslip yoga mat.

EASY POSE

Let's explore the most common sitting poses in yoga. The basic sitting posture is Easy pose. Besides being the most often used meditation posture, it is the starting position for many yoga exercises.

Sitting on a Chair

Choose a straight-backed chair with little or no padding since there can be a tendency to slump against the back of a chair. Your feet should be comfortably flat on the floor. If this is not the case, rest your feet on a firm pillow or bolster.

Sit on the floor with your legs crossed at the ankles so that your body forms a triangular base. Straighten the spine, relax the shoulders, and rest your hands on your knees. To help straighten the lower spine and allow the knees to relax down, place a firm pillow, bolster, or thick blanket under your buttocks (inset).

ROCK POSE

This pose gets its name from the idea that whoever masters Rock pose can sit and "digest rocks" since this position is beneficial for the digestive system. Rock pose also encourages a straight spine and helps you to sit as steady as a rock.

Almond oil

The almond is a wonderful nut. Its oil is excellent both internally and externally for the skin. One ounce of raw almond oil (from health-food stores), taken in food or drink each day, will help lower cholesterol, reduce body fat and hunger, cleanse the body of toxins, and keep the skin healthy and lustrous. Use instead of butter on vegetables or grains.

Sit on your heels with your feet relaxed under you. Straighten your spine. Place your hands on your thighs. To relieve excess pressure on the knees, sit with a rolled blanket or firm pillow between your buttocks and heels (right).

MUDRA

The hands form their own yoga postures, especially during meditative practices such as pranayama (breathing exercises), and sitting meditations. These hand positions, called mudras, are used to activate certain pressure points on the fingers. Each mudra is a technique for giving clear messages to the mind–body energy system.

The most common hand position is called Gyan ("ghee-yawn") mudra. This mudra activates the qualities of knowledge and wisdom (which is what *gyan* means in Sanskrit). There are two forms: passive and active.

Passive Gyan mudra
Put the tip of the thumb together with the tip of the index finger. This enhances receptivity and promotes calmness.

Active Gyan mudra
Curl the index finger under the thumb so that the fingernail is on the second joint of the thumb. This provides all the same qualities as passive Gyan Mudra but with a more active, or projective, energy.

TUNING IN

In kundalini yoga, there is a sound intonation, called a mantra, that is used to begin a yoga practice. Mantras (from the Sanskrit *man*, meaning "mind," and *tra*, meaning "guiding") are ancient, time-tested sounds that have been used to calm, focus, and uplift the mind. According to yogic understanding, and validated by science, the basic nature of everything in the universe is composed of vibration—consisting of sound, light, and energy. When chanting a mantra, every cell vibrates at a similar energy frequency in the same way that a note struck on a stringed instrument will automatically vibrate on a second instrument.

Before beginning each yoga practice, experiment with using this mantra as a centering technique to attune you to your inner guidance. *Ong Namo Guru Dev Namo* means "I call on the Universal Spirit, I call on the ever-present guidance." As you chant the mantra, feel the navel come in toward the spine slightly on the long "o" sound of *Ong*. Then feel the "ng" at the point between your two eyebrows. *Namo* is pronounced "nah-moe." *Guru* is "gu-roo"; make sure to roll the "r" sound. *Dev* sounds like "dave," and then finally *Namo* again.

The cosmic syllable *Om* is considered to be the primal sound from which all things are created. It begins with the open "o" or "au" sound, then extends the "m" sound, creating a soothing hum in the throat and root of the nose. In kundalini yoga, *Om* is changed slightly to *Ong*, which is considered to be the active form of *Om*.

To begin your practice, sit with your legs crossed, your spine straight, and bring the palms of your hands together. Press the hands into the center of your chest so that your thumbs

press against your sternum. This is called Prayer pose. Inhale deeply with your eyes closed and chant the mantra once. Repeat for a total of three repetitions.

DEEP BREATHING

To understand the mechanics of deep breathing, the most common breath used in yoga, take a look at a sleeping baby. Watch her abdomen rise effortlessly as she inhales and fall as she exhales. This is our natural, inborn way of breathing. Recognize that you have known this way of breathing and it is preserved in your cell memory. If you have forgotten how to breathe deeply, this exercise will help you retrain yourself.

Taking long, slow, deep breaths calms you, relaxes your heart, relieves stress, clears your mind, and brings awareness of your inner being.

1. Lie on your back with your knees bent. Place one hand on your abdomen and the other on your upper chest. Expel all your breath on the exhalation. Make a conscious effort to push the remaining breath out with your abdominal muscles, creating a vacuum for a deep breath to enter.

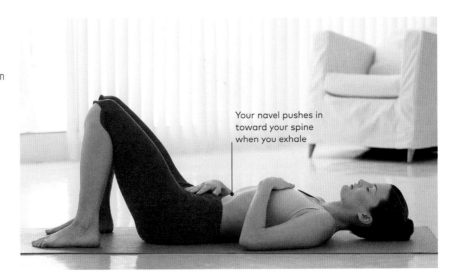

Your navel pushes in toward your spine when you exhale

2. As you begin to inhale, your abdominal muscles will relax and expand outward to allow the diaphragm to drop. Pause the breath for 1–2 seconds at the end of your inhalation. As you exhale, your abdominal muscles will naturally move inward to press the diaphragm up against the lungs. Notice the breath leaving the upper chest first. Continue exhaling smoothly and completely, and feel the abdominal muscles press slightly toward the spine. Pause the breath, then begin another deep inhalation.

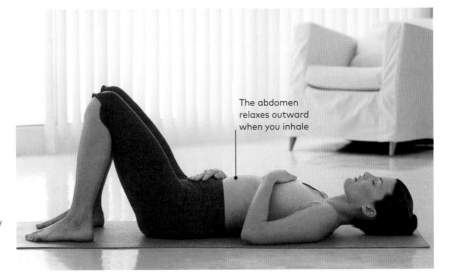

The abdomen relaxes outward when you inhale

BREATH OF FIRE

Breath of Fire is actually like one long, continuous breath being pumped in and out over and over. Because of the way it moves energy and blood circulation, there are a few cautions: during menstruation, a "light" practice of Breath of Fire will help regulate your period, but do not practice it if you have discomfort or cramping. In pregnancy, except possibly the first trimester, Breath of Fire should be avoided. If you have a major health issue, check first with your GP.

Breath of Fire cleanses the blood, the mucous linings of the lungs, and all the body cells. It rejuvenates brain neurons and expands lung capacity while strengthening all the nerves in the body.

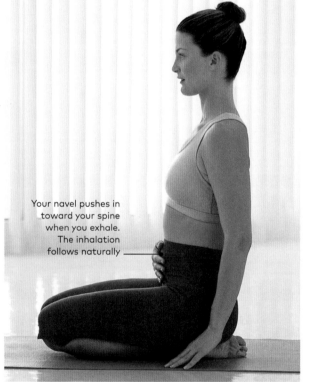

Your navel pushes in toward your spine when you exhale. The inhalation follows naturally ———

(1) Sit in Easy pose or on your heels in Rock pose. Straighten the spine and relax the shoulders. You may like to put one hand on the abdomen to monitor its movement. Inhale normally. Then exhale with force. Your navel will press back toward your spine, and you may feel the slight upward push of the diaphragm pressing the breath out of your lungs.

(2) Let the breath enter naturally on the inhalation, and press it out again on the exhalation. Although the inhalation and exhalation are equal in length, it may be helpful to focus on the strong, quick exhalation. Start off slowly, at a rate of one exhalation per 2 seconds, then as you get used to the movement, speed it up gradually so that you are exhaling at two per second or faster.

You can also contract in Root Lock on the held inhalation and release on the exhalation

ROOT LOCK

Body Locks, or Bandhas ("bond" or "tie" in Sanskrit), are internal contractions of muscles that are used to strengthen those muscles, focus concentration, and move energy through the body, which translates into vitality and health. The most commonly used lock is called Root Lock. Women who practice pelvic floor exercises will recognize the vaginal squeeze as an integral part of Root Lock.

Expel all your breath on the exhalation. Contract and lift the pelvic floor muscles, which include the anal muscles and the genitals. Try to keep the buttocks relaxed. Pull the navel in toward the spine. Hold, or lock, for a few seconds. Then as you inhale, relax the lock and focus your attention in an upward motion from the base of the spine to the top of your head. Or you may focus at the brow point (the area between your eyebrows). Exhale again and repeat several times.

Root Lock is great for certain times of a woman's life, such as the postnatal period when the internal muscles need firming and strengthening. Root Lock should not be practiced during menstruation. In cases of major health issues, check with your GP before practicing this pose.

DEEP RELAXATION

An essential part of yoga is the deep relaxation at the end of your practice. In fact, deep relaxation is actually a pose called Corpse pose. If you think this sounds morbid, think again. The idea is that you are "dead" to the world, to your bodily tensions, and to the usual cacophony of mental noise. Corpse pose is the icing on the cake of yoga practice, held dear by long-time yoga practitioners and new ones alike. In deep relaxation, you are "actively allowing" in the sense that you are consciously noticing tensions, thoughts, or feelings without giving them any extra attention; at the same time, you allow them to release. What this process does is bring you to an inner space of no resistance. In the openness of that space, the transforming power of your yoga practice can have optimum effect.

Many people, upon learning yogic deep relaxation techniques, discover that they need to relearn what it feels like to relax deeply. As your yoga practice increases, you become more aware of tension in your body and mind, and so can consciously relax yourself immediately.

(1) Lie down on a comfortably padded mat. You may want to place a rolled blanket or bolster under your knees and/or neck and cover yourself with a light, natural fabric shawl to avoid a chill (inset). If you are wearing glasses, take them off to relax the eyes. You may also like to have some beautifully uplifting music playing softly. If it is music with words, they should be elevating and divinely inspired. See Music Resources (p.224) for suggested relaxation music.

Corpse pose with shawl for added comfort.

MEDITATION SHAWL

During yoga practice, heat builds in the body to the point that you may sweat lightly. This heat rises and cools off in the period of deep relaxation or mediation that often follows a yoga practice. Covering your body with a light cotton or wool shawl during a sitting meditation is just as important as during deep relaxation: the meditation shawl not only keeps the spine warm but allows for a subtle flow of energy through the entire spine, which empowers your meditation.

2 Close your eyes. Your arms are at your sides with the palms facing upward, open and relaxed. Allow your body to feel as if it is sinking toward the floor. Consciously relax every part of your body, beginning with your feet and moving up your legs to your pelvis, torso, arms, and face (including your lips, jaw, and face muscles).

3 If your mind begins to wander, gently bring your attention back to the quiet inflow and outflow of your breath. You may like to imagine hearing a mantra or affirmation with each inhalation and exhalation. Continue to relax for at least 10 minutes, preferably longer. If you fall asleep, it will be a self-healing sleep, so light that you may feel yourself almost dancing on the edge of awareness.

COMING BACK FROM DEEP RELAXATION

At the end of your relaxation time, when you return to an awareness of yourself, take a deep and conscious inhalation and exhalation. Do the following wake-up exercises for about 20 seconds each, using deep breathing.

(1) Roll your wrists and ankles in circles in both directions. This wakes up the extremities of the body.

(2) Lift your feet and rub the bare soles together. Rub your hands together at the same time. This wakes up the nerve endings in the feet and hands.

(3) Begin a Cat Stretch: bring your arms out to the sides, straighten one leg and bring the other bent leg across it in a diagonal stretch. Turn your head in the opposite direction from your bent leg. Breathe. Then switch sides. Do this a few times on each side to give the spine and body a good diagonal stretch.

(4) Draw your knees into your chest and wrap your arms around them. Tuck your head into your chest and begin rocking up and down on your spine 6–8 times. This wakes up the spine.

(5) Sit up to end your practice or to meditate. These exercises bring your body and mind to consciousness gently and completely. Be sure to drink some spring water (room temperature) after relaxing or meditating to reground and rebalance the nervous system.

WARMING UP TO YOGA

As you leaf through this book, you'll see a wide variety of yoga sets, or kriyas, and yoga poses. Many require some flexibility and should not be done "cold." As you choose different yoga sets, refer back to this chapter for essential warm-up poses and practice them for at least 10 minutes before you move on. Choose between the Spinal Warm-ups on pp.31–37 and Kneeling Sun Salutation on pp.38–41, or do all of these for an especially satisfying experience. These exercises and poses loosen up your spine and back muscles, all the way from your tailbone to your neck. Rotating joints is key, as is stretching the nerves and muscles in the arms and legs. You will be able to accomplish all of these warm-up exercises in just 10–15 minutes.

SPINAL WARM-UPS

The following exercises prepare the body, and specifically the spine, for the rest of the yoga in this book. Although you don't need to do all of these warm-ups each time you practice yoga, the key point is to begin at the base of the spine and work your way upward toward the neck.

LOWER SPINE FLEX

In this exercise, you are loosening the vertebrae of the lower spine. The spinal fluid and pranic life energy within the lower spine are also activated and begin to circulate upward throughout the spine.

Breathing consciously is an essential aspect of yoga. Breathe deeply to expand your lung capacity, energize your brain, and oxygenate your blood. Focus on each inflow and outflow of breath for a deeper experience of peace and clarity.

① Start in Easy pose: sit on the floor with your legs crossed and tucked in. Straighten the spine by pressing the chest slightly forward and lifting the rib cage. Relax the shoulders and slightly tuck the chin in.

② Take hold of your outside ankles with both hands. Inhale and flex your spine forward. The chest lifts and the shoulders drop back. Keep your head upright as you move your spine.

③ Exhale and round the back, slump the chest, and let the shoulders fall forward. Continue in a rhythmic forward and backward manner. Feel your pelvis rock forward and back as you flex, and each vertebra of your spine curl and uncurl. Pick up the pace for 1–2 minutes, then inhale deeply, hold, exhale, and relax your breath and the pose.

UPPER SPINE FLEX

The vertebrae of the midspine are flexed in this pose, and digestion is stimulated. Energy is circulated throughout the middle and upper back. The head moves in tandem with the spine in a fluid motion.

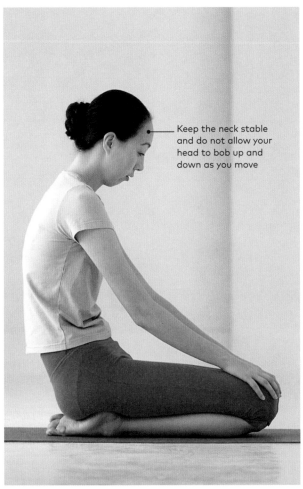

Keep the neck stable and do not allow your head to bob up and down as you move

(1) Sitting in Rock pose, place your hands on your thighs, elbows slightly bent. Inhale and stretch your body forward, hands on thighs. Your chest should be lifted, the shoulders back and relaxed, the chin slightly tucked in toward the neck.

(2) Exhale and slump the spine as far as possible, shoulders rounded forward. Keep your elbows as straight as possible throughout the exercise. Focus your awareness on the areas from the midspine up through the shoulder blades. Feel each vertebra flexing. Repeat the sequence for 1–2 minutes, beginning slowly and then picking up the pace. Inhale deeply and stretch the chest out. Then exhale and relax the breath and the pose.

TWISTS

Here, the entire spine is loosened and the vertebrae are adjusted. This active spinal twist massages all the internal organs, improves digestion, and tones the lateral and abdominal muscles.

① Sit in Easy pose (p.19), stretch the spine up, chest out, and bring your hands up to grasp the shoulders with the fingers to the front and the thumbs to the back. Keep the upper arms parallel to the ground.

② Twist as far as you can in each direction, swinging freely from side to side. Inhale to the left and exhale to the right. Breathe rhythmically and powerfully for 1–2 minutes.

HYDROTHERAPY

A brief cold shower in the morning strengthens the nervous system and opens the capillaries, flushing impurities from the bloodstream. When the capillaries return to normal, the blood supply flushes and refreshes the organs and glandular system. First, massage your body with pure oil, preferably almond; this protective coating is driven into the skin's pores while showering. Allow cold water to hit your feet, your body, and your face, but not the top of your head or thighs. Massage as you move in and out of the cold water. Breathe deeply or chant a mantra. Start with a 30-second shower, and work up to 3 minutes. Towel-dry and rub the skin briskly. If you have circulatory problems or other conditions, seek medical advice first. Pregnant and menstruating women should take warm or lukewarm showers.

SHOULDER SHRUGS

Shoulder tension is common in the fast-paced lives most of us lead, and it often contributes to tension headaches as well. In this exercise, the tension in the shoulders is pressurized as you squeeze upward and then released as you drop the shoulders.

① Sit in Easy pose. Straighten your spine and bring your neck and spinal vertebrae in line. Keep your hands relaxed on your knees. Inhale and lift your shoulders straight up.

② Exhale and let your shoulders drop down. Using a powerful breath, continue Shoulder Shrugs for 1–2 minutes. Then inhale deeply, stretch the shoulders up and hold for a few seconds, and finally exhale, relaxing down. Feel a warm energy circulating throughout the shoulder and neck area.

NECK ROLLS

In the previous exercises, spinal fluid and pranic life energy have been stimulated and circulated from the spine upward. This exercise releases the tension in the neck, allowing the energy to flow into the head.

1. Keeping your jaw relaxed and your mouth slack, gently drop your head forward, and as you inhale, begin to rotate your head around to the left shoulder. Your chin will travel over the left shoulder as you inhale and your head will slowly circle in a smooth, continuous motion.

2. As you exhale, your head will move over the right shoulder and back to the front. Move meditatively and slowly. After 3–4 circles, reverse the direction. Inhale to the right, and exhale as the head comes around to the left. Continue for 3–4 circles, then inhale and bring your head to the front. Exhale and relax.

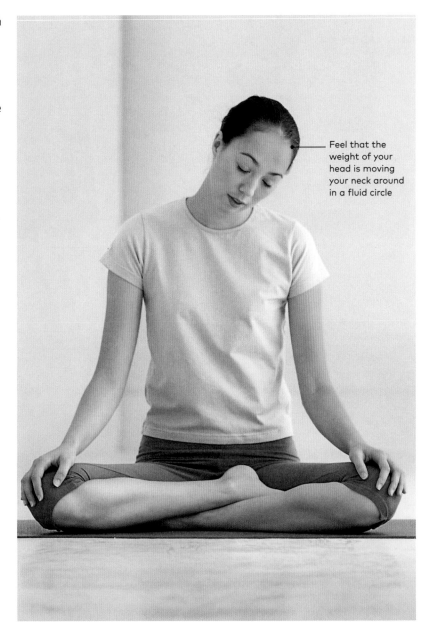

Feel that the weight of your head is moving your neck around in a fluid circle

If you have reason to be cautious about neck movements, try Neck Turns: inhale and slowly turn your head to the left, bringing your chin toward or over your shoulder, then exhale and slowly turn your head toward the right shoulder. Repeat several times.

SPREAD STRETCH

This exercise increases flexibility, stretching and strengthening the hips, lower spine, and lateral muscles from the upper chest to the pelvis. The sciatic nerve is strengthened as the leg muscles receive a beneficial stretch.

1. Spread your legs as far apart as is comfortable. Place your hands by your hips and lift your body slightly so that you are up on your buttocks and your lower spine is straight.

2. Inhale as you stretch your arms straight up overhead, lengthening the spine and lifting the rib cage.

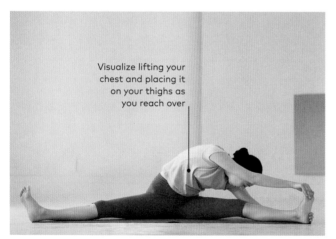

Visualize lifting your chest and placing it on your thighs as you reach over

3. Exhale and reach for the outside of your left foot with your left hand and for the left toes with your right hand. If you cannot reach this far, hold your ankle or calf. Keep your chin parallel to the ground. Inhale and lift up to the center.

4. Exhale and stretch over your right leg in the same manner as for the left leg. Inhale and lift up to the center again. Continue this stretching sequence for 1–2 minutes.

5 Inhale and lift up to the center, then exhale down. Stretch your hands out toward each ankle and bring your chest close to the floor, lengthening the spine as you do so. Hold this downward stretch and begin either deep breathing or Breath of Fire for 1 minute. Then inhale and hold the breath for a few seconds.

6 Exhale and slowly sit up. Use your hands to push up from the ground to bring yourself back to a sitting position and avoid straining the lower back.

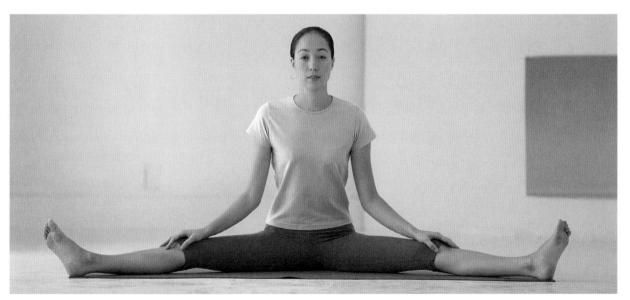

7 Inhale deeply as you return to the upright position. Then exhale and relax out of the position. Only stretch as much as feels comfortable in this exercise if you are not flexible.

KNEELING SUN SALUTATION

This series of postures is a modified version of the classic Sun Salutation. By regularly practicing the Kneeling Sun Salutation, you will find it easier to practice the Moon Salutation (p.79). The Kneeling Sun Salutation will flex your spine in every direction, stretch your limbs, deepen your breathing, and enable you to experience a place of peace.

When you move from one posture into another in a set—inhaling into one pose, exhaling into the next, and so on—the set is referred to as Vinyasa. This dynamic style of yoga practice allows your body to get used to the postures gently and gradually. As you move, the Vinyasa allows you to focus your breath on different parts of your body and heighten the intensity of the effect of each movement. Once you get a feel for it, it becomes a beautiful yoga dance of your body and your breathing.

As you become familiar with moving body and breath together in a Vinyasa, you can add in other poses at certain points. For example, add Upward Facing Dog (step 6) after Downward Dog (step 5) in this set.

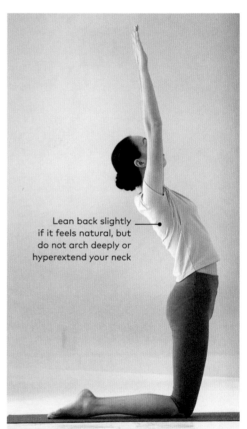

Lean back slightly if it feels natural, but do not arch deeply or hyperextend your neck

① Sit back on your heels in Rock pose (p.20) and place your hands on your thighs. If this is uncomfortable, kneel up so that your body forms a straight line from the knees upward.

② As you inhale, kneel upright slowly and lift your arms out in front of your body, then extend them upward. As you complete your inhalation, stretch fully up with your chest lifted and arms extended overhead. Pause the breath for a few seconds. For those with lower back pain, sweep your arms out to the sides of your body first and then up.

Pause briefly at the end of each movement to maintain your awareness of your body movements

③ As you begin to exhale, slowly sit back on the heels once again while you bring your arms back down in front of your body. As you near the end of your exhalation, dome the back and bring your forehead to the ground in an extended Child's pose, with your arms stretched out in front of you on the ground. Hold the exhale and remain still for a few seconds. To protect your lower back, sit back onto the heels before bringing the arms down just in front of your knees. Then as you bring your forehead to the ground, stretch your arms out in front of you and finish the exhale.

④ Inhale and lean into your arms as you lift your body forward onto your knees and hands with your buttocks up. Your spine curves toward the ground and your head is lifted with the shoulders relaxed. Lengthen your spine and press the tailbone back as you complete the inhalation. This is called Cow pose.

⑤ As you exhale, keep the hands in place while you come onto your feet and hands in Downward Dog. Your body forms a triangle with your buttocks at the highest point. Straighten the legs and press the heels to the ground. Stretch your spine away from the ground. Your hips will move toward the ceiling and back away from your hands. This will give your arms, spine, and legs a deep stretch. ▶

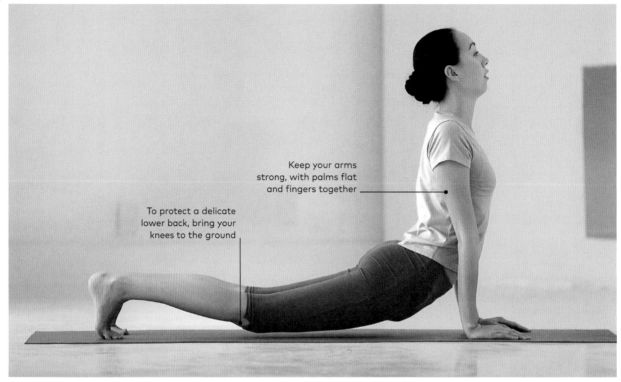

Keep your arms strong, with palms flat and fingers together

To protect a delicate lower back, bring your knees to the ground

⑥ Either go on to step 8 or move into Upward Facing Dog: position your feet a few inches farther back as you begin inhaling. Lower your body down until it is a few inches from the ground.

Press into your arms and lift your chest and head in Upward Facing Dog pose as you finish the inhalation. Keep your movements fluid.

⑦ Exhale as you return to Downward Dog (step 5), lifting the pelvis upward and pressing it back. You may need to adjust your feet again, bringing them forward a few steps.

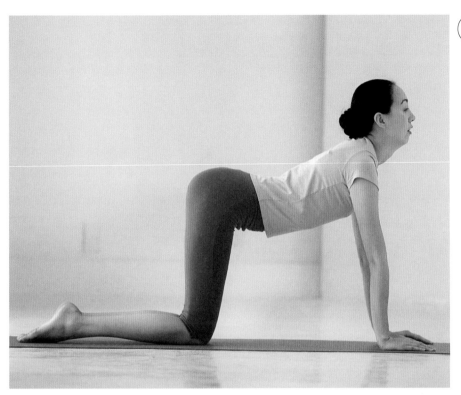

⑧ Begin to reverse the order of the Vinyasa: as you inhale, gently come onto your knees into Cow pose (step 4).

⑨ Exhale back into the extended Child's pose, following the sequence described in step 3.

⑩ Inhale and exhale into Rock pose—back to step 1—to end one round of Kneeling Sun Salutation. Inhale and repeat the sequence from step 2 for as many rounds as you like.

STRENGTHEN & INVIGORATE

All yoga is good for women—as for men—but some poses especially resonate with the physical and mental makeup of women. As a woman, it is imperative for your health and happiness that you exercise every day. If you begin to find yourself feeling moody or easily frazzled, you need to move your body! This helps move your mind into new and brighter places. The poses explored here can all be practiced with either deep breathing or Breath of Fire. Some women like to practice them as a daily routine, while others prefer to add a few as warm-ups before a yoga set or spontaneously practice a few postures in between busy moments in the day. Whatever your method, you will experience an increase in strength, rejuvenation, and relaxation from these poses.

CAT AND COW STRETCH

This exercise brings increased flexibility to the spine, including the cervical vertebrae, and circulates the spinal fluid. A great warm-up exercise, Cat and Cow will prepare you for the other postures in this chapter.

(1) Position yourself on your hands and knees, with your knees under your hips and your hands under your shoulders. As far as possible, keep your elbows straight and your arms and legs stable throughout the exercise as your spine curves in each direction.

(2) As you inhale, arch the spine toward the ground and bring your head back into Cow pose.

(3) As you exhale, flex in the opposite direction so that your back is arched upward and your head comes down so that your chin is close to your chest. This is Cat pose. Alternate between Cat and Cow poses for 2–3 minutes, gradually increasing the speed and the power of each breath as you continue.

LIFE NERVE STRETCH

In yogic teachings, your sciatic nerve is also called your life nerve.
Keeping your life nerve strong and stretched is important for
the health and flexibility of your body.

① Sit high on your buttocks with your legs stretched out in front of you, your arms by your sides with palms flat and fingers facing forward.

② Keep your left leg straight or slightly to the side. Tuck the right foot into the groin, the heel as close to the top of the inner thigh as is comfortable. Inhale and stretch your arms up to lengthen the spine.

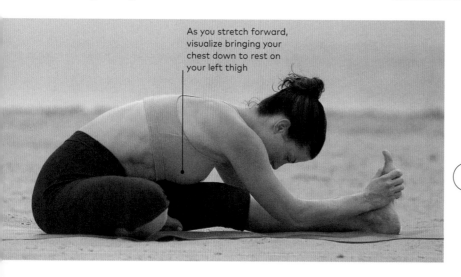

As you stretch forward, visualize bringing your chest down to rest on your left thigh

③ Exhale and bend forward, cupping your hands around your foot or holding any part of the leg that you can reach to give you a good stretch without straining. Hold the posture and breathe deeply for 1–2 minutes. Repeat on the other leg.

LOCUST

This exercise strengthens the lower back; allows energy to flow to the spine; opens the nerve channels in the solar plexus; and tones the legs, buttocks, and stomach. It stretches and massages the abdominal and reproductive organs, stimulating the digestive process. This exercise may be helpful to ease the uncomfortable bloating that can be experienced premenstrually.

(1) Lie on your stomach with your heels close together and your chin on the ground. Make fists of your hands and tuck them into the spot where they fit comfortably just inside the pelvic bones (where the legs and pelvis meet). Your hands will act as a fulcrum for raising your legs.

Use your thigh, abdominal, and lower back muscles to raise your legs

(2) Inhale and raise your legs as straight and as high as possible. Begin deep breathing for 1–3 minutes. If you have back problems, raise one leg at a time and hold for at least 15 seconds as you breathe.

(3) Relax down, bringing your arms to rest at your sides and turning your head to one side. Breathe deeply for a few moments.

BOW

This posture massages and invigorates the internal organs, strengthens the abdominal muscles, and expands your breathing capacity. It helps to prevent digestive and bowel disorders and reduces fat around the waist area. Bow pose also stretches the thigh muscles, which—according to yogic teachings—controls the calcium–magnesium balance in the body. This balance is necessary for both physical and mental well-being.

Chest-opening poses help to strengthen the lungs and, alongside conventional treatments, can support the management of conditions such as asthma. Bow creates a strong opening for the chest, enhancing lung capacity.

1   Lie on your abdomen with your chin on the ground and arms resting at your sides.

2   Bend your right leg at the knee. Reach back with your right hand and grasp the right ankle.

3   Bend your left leg at the knee and reach back with your left hand to grasp the left ankle.

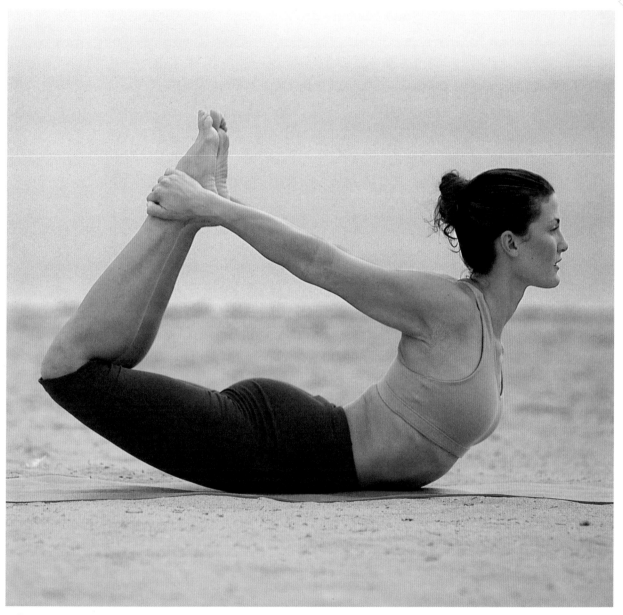

(4) Inhale and lift your body upward, raising your head, chest, and thighs off the ground. Create a tension between your straight arms and your legs to stretch higher. Breathe deeply, expanding the chest on the inhale and relaxing it on the exhale. Relax, then repeat, continuing in this way for 1–2 minutes.

Easy-does-it-version

If you can't reach your ankles, use a prop such as a belt around the ankles to grasp onto. If you can reach them but can't stretch and hold, inhale as you stretch up and exhale as you relax down. With steady practice, you will be able to do the full pose.

CAMEL

This pose builds strength in the muscle groups of the back, helping to prevent sciatica and slipped discs. Camel pose also helps to balance the navel chakra, which is your energy center of personal health and willpower, and relieves the stomach from the effects of overeating. According to yogic teaching, whoever does Camel pose regularly has control over hunger and thirst, just as a camel would. Like Bow, Camel pose also stretches the thigh muscles to control the calcium–magnesium balance in the body that is needed for both physical and mental well-being.

Golden milk

This is wonderful for the spine, lubricates the joints, and helps to break up calcium deposits. Boil ¼–⅓ tsp turmeric in ⅓ cup water for 8 minutes. Add 1 cup milk and 1 tbsp raw almond oil. Remove from heat at boiling point and add honey to taste.

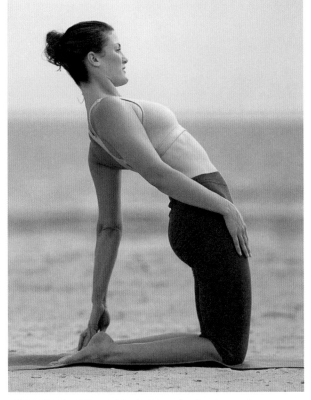

① Sit on your heels in Rock pose (p.20), with your spine straight and hands on your thighs.

② Kneel upright, reach back with one hand, and grasp the heel on that side. Repeat on the other side.

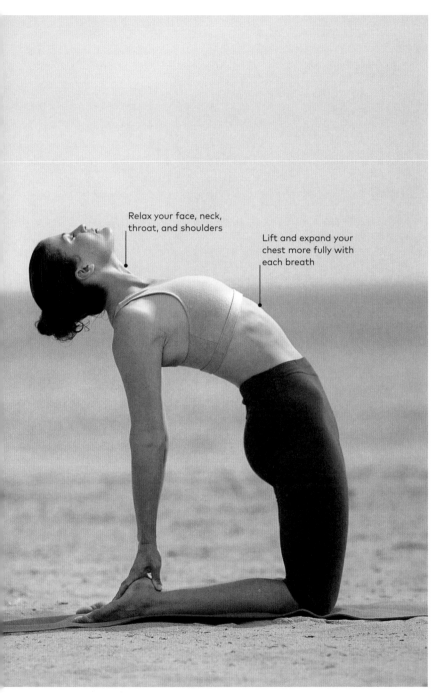

Relax your face, neck, throat, and shoulders

Lift and expand your chest more fully with each breath

③ Press the hips and thighs forward to steady the pose and to create a deeper stretch. The chest is lifted up and the head is tipped back but not dropped fully. Relax your face, neck, throat, and shoulders. Breathe deeply or use Breath of Fire (p.24) for 1–2 minutes.

Easy-does-it version

① Sit on your heels in Rock pose with your spine straight.

② Lean back onto your hands, keeping the chest lifted. Point your fingers either toward or away from your body.

③ Lift your buttocks off the ground as high as possible as you press the hips and thighs forward. Continue for 1–2 minutes.

CHILD'S POSE

Child's pose is a resting pose that allows the effects of previous yoga exercises to be assimilated. Pressing your forehead to the floor activates the sixth (intuitive) center between the eyebrows. Child's pose also acts as a counterpose to Bow pose (pp.46–47), relaxing and curving the spine in the opposite direction. If needed, add a small pillow or rolled towel under the head or under the buttocks for comfort in this pose.

Yogi tea

This health-promoting drink is delicious and a great coffee substitute. The spices used are particularly beneficial to internal health.

To 2 quarts of water, add:
15 whole cloves
20 green cardamom pods
(crushed slightly)
15 black peppercorns
5 × 2-in (5-cm) sticks cinnamon
or 8 slices ginger root
Cover and boil gently for 30–40 minutes
(adding water as it evaporates). Add
½ tsp black tea and 3–4 cups organic milk
(dairy or nondairy). Bring to a boil, then
turn off the heat and add honey to taste.

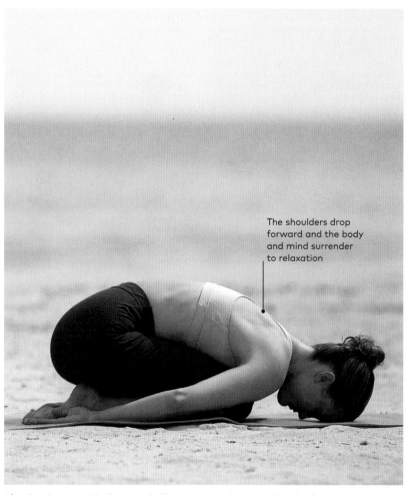

The shoulders drop forward and the body and mind surrender to relaxation

After Camel pose (pp.48–49), rest in Child's pose. Rest your buttocks on your heels and bring your forehead to the ground and your arms alongside your body, with the palms facing upward in a relaxed manner. Breathe gently for 1–2 minutes, relaxing the entire spine and shoulders.

STRETCH POSE

Stretch pose is known to adjust and balance your navel point, which increases stamina, willpower, and well-being. When your navel point is strong and balanced, you have a steady pulse centered at the navel—not left, right, above, or below it. You can check your navel pulse by bringing the thumb and fingers of one hand together and pressing deep into the skin surrounding the navel. As an experiment, check your pulse beforehand, then again immediately after this pose, practicing Stretch pose for 1–2 minutes, and notice what differences you discover. Generally, your pulse will be deeper, stronger, and more evenly centered at the navel point after practicing Stretch pose.

According to yogic tradition, the navel is the focal point for all 72,000 nerves in the body. So Stretch pose tunes up the whole nervous system, as well as the digestive and reproductive systems.

① Tuck your pelvis forward to take any pressure off the lower spine before coming up into Stretch pose. This will help to ensure that when you lift your legs up, it will be your abdominal muscles rather than your back muscles that are supporting your lift. Before lifting your head, consciously relax your neck muscles and prepare to use your upper back, chest, and abdominal muscles to lift your neck and head. This will avoid straining your neck in any way.

② Keep your heels close together and raise them 6 in (15 cm) from the ground with straight legs. Raise your head 6 in (15 cm) and fix your eyes on your pointed toes. Stay mindful of keeping the neck and lower spine relaxed while holding the pose. Your arms are held at your sides, palms facing the thighs but not touching. Hold this position for 1–2 minutes while doing Breath of Fire (p.24). Then relax down for a few seconds.

SHOULDERSTAND

Shoulderstand is said to benefit the entire body, especially the throat, thyroid, and circulation. Shoulderstand increases flexibility in the cervical region of the spine and helps prevent varicose veins. The muscles of the back, shoulders, and arms are stretched and strengthened, too. It also provides an inverted gravitational pull, which suspends and relaxes all your internal organs. Make sure you read through all the instructions before attempting this pose.

Shoulderstand inversion is one of the most powerful asanas with benefits for the whole body, particularly the throat and circulation. Increased blood flow to the throat may nourish the thyroid and improve function, while varicose veins may be prevented or limited as gravity encourages efficient blood flow back to the heart.

(1) Lie on your back with your legs bent at the knees and your feet flat on the ground. Your arms are at your sides with your palms facing downward.

(2) Keeping your arms and hands in the same position, raise your legs to a 90° angle.

USING PROPS IN SHOULDERSTAND

To relieve pressure on the neck area in Shoulderstand, place one or two thick felt blankets under your shoulders and upper back, just at the edge where your shoulders meet your neck. The blanket should be large enough so that you can also rest your elbows on it and feel stable. Your neck will then have room to relax and straighten when you come up into Shoulderstand. Another alternative and good preparation for Shoulderstand is found in Pelvic Tilt Position 2 (p.64).

After Shoulderstand, rest on your back
for a minute or two, either with your
legs out straight or, if there is pressure
on the lower spine, with your knees
bent and your pelvis tipped slightly
forward, or put a firm pillow
under your knees.

③ Begin to push your body up. Bend
your knees over your face, then
straighten your legs as much as
possible while supporting your back
with your hands and your elbows,
which remain firmly on the ground.

④ Relax and stretch up higher on your
shoulders. Adjust your hand positions:
the farther your hands move toward
your upper back, the straighter your
spine will be. Your chin should rest on
your chest. Breathe evenly as you hold
for 1–2 minutes.

⑤ To come out of the pose, lower your legs over your head
into a modified Plow pose, keeping your knees close to
your head. As you roll out slowly, place your arms on the
floor beside you, or continue to support your spine with
your hands on your back. Exhale deeply.

ARCHER

Archer pose develops the quality of courage in the face of a challenge. It balances and strengthens the nervous system and your electromagnetic energy field, or aura. Every one of your chakras is activated in this pose: the leg position works on the first, second, and third chakras; the stretch across the chest and the arm positions work to activate the heart center; and the turned neck stimulates the throat chakra. The gazing and strong breathing work on the intuitive (sixth) center and the crown center.

Archer pose calls forth the spirit of the fearless warrior. As you hold the final inhalation and stretch into the posture, visualize energy rising from the root chakra up through all the chakras. Project that energy through your gaze.

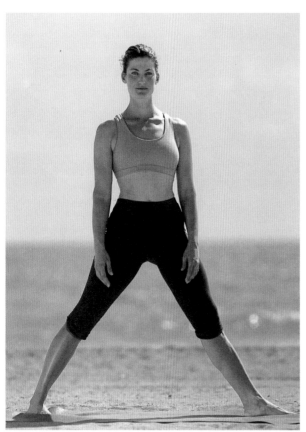

① Stand with your legs straddled about 30 in (75 cm) apart, with your left leg forward, foot turned to the side, and your right leg back at a 45° angle to the front foot. The right foot should face forward.

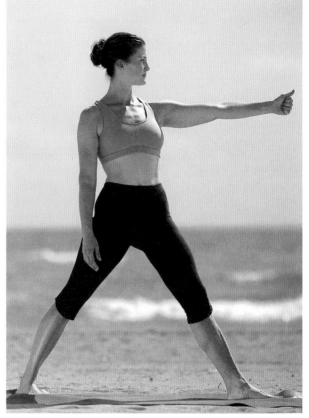

② Raise your left arm straight out in front, parallel to the ground, and make a fist as if grasping a bow while pressing the thumb forward. Turn your head to face forward and fix your eyes above your fist on the horizon.

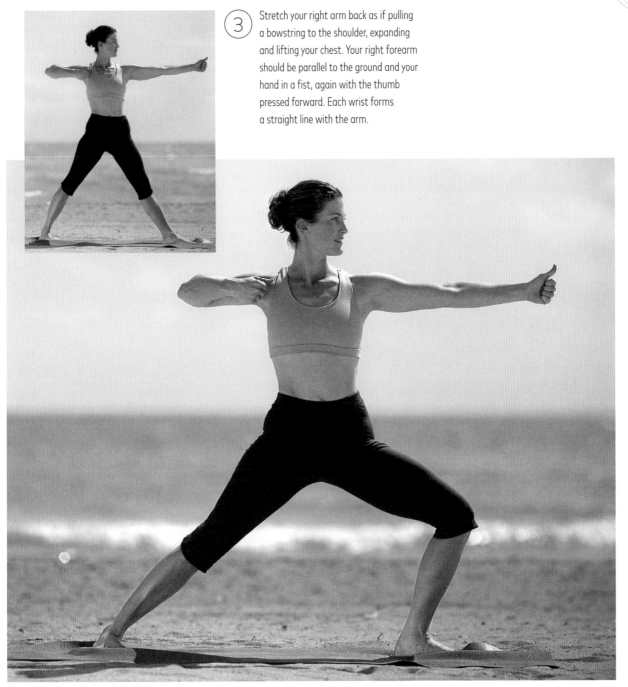

3 Stretch your right arm back as if pulling a bowstring to the shoulder, expanding and lifting your chest. Your right forearm should be parallel to the ground and your hand in a fist, again with the thumb pressed forward. Each wrist forms a straight line with the arm.

4 Bend your left knee and lean into it so that you cannot see your left foot. Keep your body centered, and without leaning forward, put 70 percent of your weight on the front leg. Begin deep, full, slow breaths or Breath of Fire. After 1–2 minutes, inhale deeply, then exhale and lean into the pose as fully as you are able to without straining. Relax and switch legs.

SAT KRIYA

This kriya, or set, practiced with the chant Sat Nam (p.16), strengthens and balances the entire sexual system and eliminative system. Your general physical health is improved because all the internal organs receive a gentle rhythmic massage from this exercise. Beginners should practice Sat Kriya for 1 minute, slowly working up to 3 minutes. After a time of steady practice, the period of Sat Kriya can be extended, and it is good to practice every day for at least 3 minutes. However, remember to approach this powerful kriya with respect. Ideally, you should relax for at least the same amount of time as you have practiced Sat Kriya, and it is recommended that you relax for up to twice that amount of time.

Yoga can help enhance women's sexual satisfaction. Sat Kriya gently massages the internal organs and strengthens the pelvic floor, which may improve sexual and reproductive health.

(1) Sit in Rock pose. Place your hand on your abdomen and pull the navel up and in toward the spine while saying *Sat*. Your breath will go out as you chant. Then take a very quick and short inhalation through your mouth as you relax your abdomen. Then chant *Nam* and begin again. Practice this step the first few times you try Sat Kriya to learn the internal movement. After that, begin step 2.

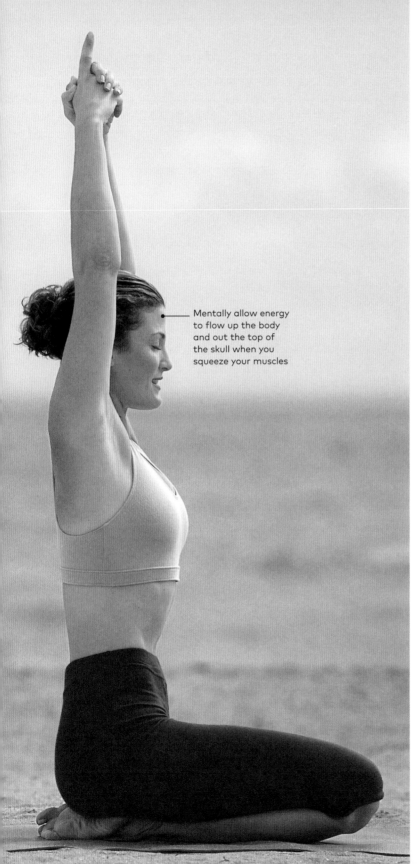

Mentally allow energy
to flow up the body
and out the top of
the skull when you
squeeze your muscles

② Stretch your arms up straight so that they are
close to the sides of your head. Interlace all the
fingers except the index fingers of each hand,
which point straight up. Say *Sat* as you pull the
navel up and *Nam* as you relax the belly area
for 1–3 minutes. Then inhale and squeeze
the muscles tightly from the buttocks, up
the back, and past the shoulders. Hold for
5–10 seconds. Exhale and relax.

③ After Sat Kriya, rest in Gurpranam pose, with
the arms positioned in front of you and the
palms of your hands together in Prayer pose.
This is a pose of surrender and devotion. You
may also rest in Child's pose (p.50) or on
your back in Corpse pose (pp.26–27) for a
period of time.

The chant, *Sat Nam*, means "truth-
identity," or "Truth is my essence."
Chant in a constant rhythm about once
a second. *Sat* should be said powerfully
but not necessarily loud. *Nam* is short,
the syllable is not extended, and it may
be barely audible.

RELAXING & ENERGIZING

Experience the freedom and joy that is grounded in a steady yoga practice and a meditative mind. From this expansive vantage point, you are open to all the possibilities that life has to offer.

How does yoga accomplish this? Yoga fosters awareness. Through yoga, you become aware of tension in your body and discord in your mind. You practice relaxing and releasing yoga. Or when you are tired and your mind is clouded, you choose yoga to bring physical energy and mental clarity. Eventually you'll be amazed to discover that yoga provides a deeply satisfying balance of true relaxation and, at the same time, an uplifting sense of energy.

REJUVENATING YOGA

We have amazing powers of self-regeneration. Our challenge is to believe in our innate capacity to rebalance, and to achieve this with integrity and without guilt. When we are frazzled at the end of the day, we know what will renew us—a few minutes of quiet time, a walk in the woods, a good book and a bath, or a small, candle-lit sanctuary for yoga. This chapter—and to a great degree, this book—is designed to foster the self-regenerating capacity of woman through yoga. Here, you will have the chance to unwind the tight muscles of your body and the restrictive pressures of your mind through restorative yoga, wall yoga, and a yogic technique called Alternate Nostril Breathing.

RESTORATIVE YOGA

Sometimes we need to stop doing and just be. That's when restorative yoga comes to the rescue. These soothing, calming poses encourage your own natural healing processes to activate, whether to help relieve stress, back pain, high blood pressure, asthma, or any number of imbalances. The poses are wonderful tools for support and relaxation during menstruation and menopause.

Suggested props

• **Bolster** A cotton-filled cushion with round ends. A thick blanket or couch cushion may be substituted.

• **Blanket** One or more firmly pressed felt-type wool or cotton blankets.

• **Eyebag** To relax the face and eyes. A folded washcloth may be substituted.

BASIC RELAXATION

This helps lower blood pressure and heart rate, releases muscular tension, reduces fatigue, improves sleep, and enhances the immune response. Use a bolster and rolled towel; an eyebag and blanket for warmth are optional.

Your chin should be slightly lower than your forehead

Make sure that you feel completely at ease and supported by your props

Lie down and place the rolled towel in the curve of your neck so that it fits comfortably. This position calms the frontal lobes of the brain. If you have tension in your lower back, place a bolster under your knees.

Make sure your legs are relaxed and your knees are supported. If your heels do not touch the floor, place a folded blanket under them.

If you are using an extra blanket for warmth, pull that over you now, and if you have an eyebag, cover your eyes with it. Lie in Corpse pose. If you are more than three months pregnant, practice Side-lying pose (p.183).

SIMPLE SUPPORTED BACKBEND

This is a welcome remedy for the common habit of slouching forward. The muscles of the middle and upper back stretch and relax, the rib cage is opened, and all the organs of the upper body are rejuvenated. You will need a bolster and, if extra support is needed, one or two blankets and a towel.

Do not practice if you have lower back pain, disc disease, are more than three months pregnant, or menstruating.

(1) If you need neck support, roll a blanket or towel in a way that will maintain the natural curve of your neck. Position a bolster where your middle back will lie and place a rolled blanket under your shoulders at a comfortable height. Bend your knees or place a rolled blanket under them to protect your back and relax the abdomen. Rest your arms on the floor above your head or out to the side, whichever is comfortable. Stay in the pose for up to 1 minute, gradually increasing the time.

(2) Roll to one side and remove any props from under your neck and shoulders.

(3) Remove the bolster and rest your lower back flat on the ground for a few breaths.

SUPPORTED CHILD'S POSE

This gently stretches the lower back, eases tension in the abdomen, relieves shoulder tension, and quiets the mind. It is a good counterpose for backbends. Do not practice this if you have a chronic back condition or are more than three months pregnant.

You will need a bolster or a few blankets for stacking. If desired, use a blanket to cover yourself with.

1 Kneel on a mat with your knees apart and your bolster between your thighs. To avoid stressing the ligaments of your outer ankles, point your toes backward, not toward each other. To take pressure off the knee joints, place a rolled towel toward the bend in the knees.

The counterpressure of the bolster may feel especially good if you have menstrual cramps or trapped air in the intestines

2 Rest your chest gently on the bolster. If you need more height, add a blanket or pillow to the bolster. Let your tailbone drop toward your heels to lengthen your lower back as you relax. Turn your head to each side for a minute or so. Your arms may either reach back toward your feet or forward around the edges of the bolster. Close your eyes. Practice for 2–3 minutes.

3 When you come out of the pose, stretch your legs forward and massage or shake your legs, especially around your knees, before you stand up.

WALL YOGA

For each of these exercises, prepare your space by placing a yoga mat and/or a felt blanket on the ground up close to the edge of the wall. The mat should be long enough to fit your body and head. Do not practice these postures if you are more than three months pregnant.

PELVIC TILTS

As you straighten up and curl down, you will feel a "rubber band" stretch in the body. The floor provides support for the spine, as well as a gentle massage to individual vertebra as you curl and uncurl the spine.

Position One
Lie on the mat with your buttocks about 12 in (30 cm) from the wall. Bend your knees and place your feet on the wall around 18 in (45 m) from the base of the wall. Place your arms on the ground at your sides, palms facing downward. Inhale and lift the torso slightly off the ground, leading with your pelvis, and bend your knees toward the wall (inset). Your spine will automatically straighten and lengthen. Exhale and reverse the motion.

Position Two
Lie on the mat so that your buttocks are 12 in (30 cm) from the wall. Place your feet 3½ ft (1.1 m) up on the wall, about 8 in (20 cm) apart and parallel with each other. Inhale and lift the pelvis and torso high so that you are in a modified Shoulderstand (inset). Press your hands against the ground. Hold the position for five deep breaths. Slowly roll down on the exhale: begin to curve the upper spine toward the ground, then the lower spine.

NECK HELPER

This exercise trains your back, chest, and abdominal muscles to support the lifting of your head. In this way, you avoid strain and your neck muscles are strengthened in the process.

(1) Lie on the mat so that your buttocks are about 12 in (30 cm) from the wall. Bend your knees and place your feet on the wall around 18 in (45 cm) from the base of the wall. Place your arms on the ground at your sides with the palms facing downward.

(2) As you exhale, begin to lift the chest, allowing the head to follow. Relax your neck and feel that your head is lifted by your upper body muscles. This allows the neck to lift without strain. Then inhale and lower your upper chest and neck, with the chest and back muscles supporting the neck.

YOGURT BATH

For relaxing your body and nourishing your skin, take a yogurt bath. This is especially beneficial following menstruation—a time for pampering yourself. Light a candle and have some soft, relaxing music playing. Warm up plain yogurt (preferably homemade) and steam up the bathroom first so that the bathtub is warm. Sit in the empty bathtub and massage yogurt all over your body, including your hair and scalp if you wish. Take your time, breathe slowly, and consciously relax. Continue for between 15 minutes and an hour, then rinse off the yogurt in a warm shower. Lie down and relax for up to one hour.

TAILOR

This resting pose aligns and supports the spine, hips, and buttocks. The hips and pelvis relax and open fully, and the thighs stretch and open as the knees gently press toward the wall. Do not practice this pose if you are more than three months pregnant.

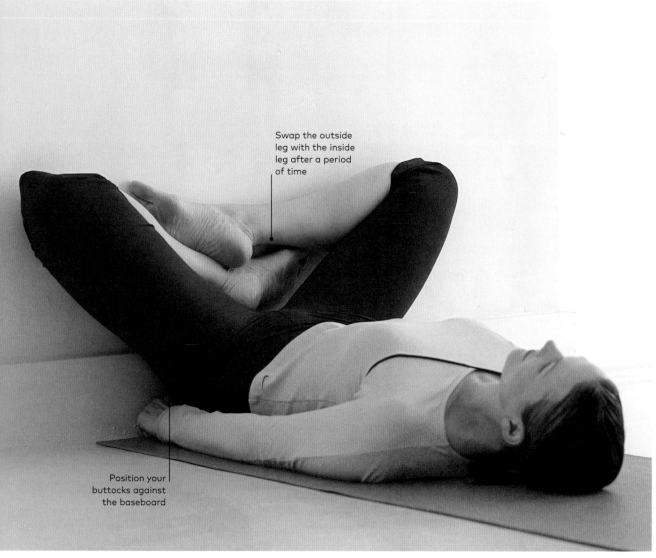

Swap the outside leg with the inside leg after a period of time

Position your buttocks against the baseboard

Lie on the ground with the buttocks against the baseboard of the wall. Cross your legs and tuck one foot toward the inside of your thigh. The other foot rests to the outside of your tucked leg. Continue for 1–3 minutes, then switch the inside and outside leg position to balance the hips.

STRENGTHENING INNER THIGHS

This strengthens the nervous system and the inner thigh muscles, which are often weak and easily injured. Do this slowly, with conscious awareness of activating the thigh muscles. Do not practice this pose if you are more than three months pregnant.

1. With your buttocks against the baseboard, straighten the legs against the wall. Consciously activate the inner thigh muscles by imagining you are hugging the muscle to the bone. You may feel a slight stiffening in the thigh muscles as you do this.

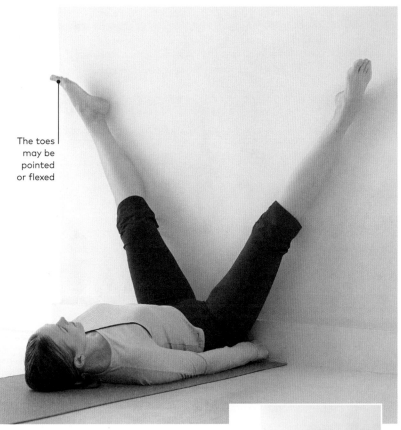

The toes may be pointed or flexed

2. Begin to inhale and open the legs slowly to around 3 ft (1 m) wide, controlling the movement with the thigh muscles. As you slowly exhale, take 5 seconds to slowly bring the legs back together. Repeat 5–10 times.

3. After this exercise, close your knees with your feet against the wall and hug your knees to your chest for a few seconds.

ENDING WALL YOGA

Knowing how to move away from the wall when you are finished is important. The muscles and joints that you have exercised and stretched may be in a delicate state, so it is best to move slowly and follow the three steps below.

① Bring your knees to one side and roll your body down onto that side. Steady yourself with one hand.

② Making a smooth transition from step 1, come up onto your hands and knees.

③ You may like to counter-stretch for a minute in Child's pose, with your forehead on the ground and your arms relaxed on the floor by your sides.

PRACTICING ALTERNATE NOSTRIL BREATHING

According to yogic teachings, nostrils are gateways to vast energy within the body. The left nostril cools the air as it is drawn in, which relaxes you. The right nostril warms the air as it draws it in, energizing you. Breathe through one nostril at a time to calm or energize yourself.

(1) Sit with a straight spine. Using the right hand, extend the thumb, ring finger, and little finger. Fold the index finger and middle finger toward your palm. Block the right nostril with your thumb. Inhale through the left nostril.

In yogic science, the left side of the body is the moon side: cooling, receptive, feminine energy. The right side is the sun side: warming, projective, masculine energy.

(2) After you have inhaled, and your thumb is still gently pressing against your right nostril, bring your ring finger onto your left nostril so that both nostrils are now closed. Hold them closed for a few seconds.

(3) To exhale, lift your thumb and exhale through your right nostril. Empty your lungs, and begin again, inhaling through your right nostril and exhaling through your left nostril. Repeat for 5 minutes.

TO RELAX & REJOICE

It's easy to feel like rejoicing when you are relaxed. So getting relaxed is the first step—always. Take relaxation breaks throughout the day, even if they last for only a couple of minutes. Excuse yourself from your work and move outdoors or into a private room for a few minutes of quiet where you can hear yourself breathe and feel your body unwind as tension falls away. Strong exercise and breathing automatically lead to relaxation by releasing tension stored in the body. Whether you prefer working out, jogging, or free-form dance, moving your body releases stress, and that is exactly what we will explore in the creative yoga practice contained in this part of the book.

MOVEMENT RELAXATION

Rhythmic, unforced, graceful, and free movement relaxes the entire body and mind, releasing everyday emotional traumas that leave their signature of tension in the body. If these areas are not relaxed, built-up stress can lead to physical and mental health imbalances. This simple set of yoga exercises, enhanced by meditative music, is a lovely self-expression and self-healing modality.

1 MOVEMENT

In the first part of this exercise, you draw your awareness into your inner body. Then, as you dance from a place of inner awareness, your body and mind work as one. Use music (p.224) for steps 1 and 2, or just step 2.

(1) Stand up straight with your arms completely relaxed. Close your eyes. Become aware of each part of your body from the inside, starting with the feet and slowly working up to your head. Allow the tension to release in each part. Consciously let it go.

(2) Keeping your eyes closed, begin to dance, swaying and moving each body part. Move in whichever way you want to. Express yourself through the movement of your body, continuing for 3–11 minutes or as long as you like.

2 TOUCH

Feeling the entire body confirms the reality of the relaxation, is self-healing, and smooths the aura (the energy field surrounding you).

Balance

My viniyoga teacher has taught me much about balance: "Be like a deer in a forest. She stops, listens, feels. The deer is very still, at ease, yet alert. Everything is coming into her field of sensations and awareness. Watch the interplay between expanded awareness while being at ease, and you will understand the two essential elements of yoga: *sukhum* (ease) and *sthiram* (alertness)."

Feel sensitively with the palms of your hands and bless yourself with your touch

Stand straight with eyes closed. With your hands, begin to lightly feel each part of your body without reservation, not forgetting the soles of the feet and the backs of the hands. Continue for 2–5 minutes.

3 FORWARD & BACKWARD HANG

The last exercise in this set strengthens the heart and circulatory system. If this system is weak, tissues in the extremities and in the joints may build up deposits that can lead to illness.

Poses that bring the head below the heart help to relieve stress and support cardiovascular health.

① Lean forward with arms completely relaxed and hanging down. Keep the knees relaxed and unlocked. Allow every muscle in your body to relax. Let your breath be relaxed and natural. Stay in this position for 2–11 minutes.

② Inhale and exhale deeply several times, then slowly straighten up. Take 30 seconds to 1 minute to return to an upright position.

③ In a continuous motion, slowly lean backward with arms hanging loosely. For neck problems, tip the head back only as far as is comfortable. Hold for 1 minute, then slowly straighten your body and completely relax.

YOGA TO HELP YOU SLEEP

Sleeplessness has become a major problem in our society. In general, a practice of yoga will do wonders for relaxing the body and mind in preparation for sleep. Do the following exercises before bed or anytime that sleep has been interrupted. Feel free to practice these together or individually. You may like to add in some relaxing poses from Rejuvenating Yoga (pp.60–69).

TABLE

This posture opens the pathway for the spinal fluid to circulate to the brain as it strengthens the nervous system. It promotes deep relaxation through the tensing of muscles and the subsequent release of tension in the arms, neck, legs, and abdomen.

1 Lie down on your back. Bend your knees and put your feet flat on the ground and your arms at your sides.

2 Keeping your knees bent, sit up. Lean back slightly while keeping your chest lifted. Place your hands on the ground behind you with the fingers pointing inward if possible.

(3) Push yourself up into Table pose. Your body forms a straight line from your head to your knees. Your neck is in line with the rest of your body and is not dropped fully back. Begin Breath of Fire or deep breathing for 1–3 minutes.

(4) Lower your buttocks back down to the floor as in step 2, then relax on your back and rest for a few seconds.

TENSION RELEASER

In this exercise, a strong tension is created, then released all at once. It strengthens the nervous system, releases built-up tension, and is excellent to do before going to bed. The more tension you can put into the action, the deeper your relaxation will be afterward.

Open your fingers wide, then close them tightly, as though you are grasping something

(1) Lie down comfortably on your back. Mentally relax every part of your body. Inhale and reach to the sky with your arms and hands.

Keep the rest of your body relaxed

(2) While creating as much tension as possible in your arms, hands, face, and upper chest, slowly pull your hands toward your chest. Let your arms shake. Hold your breath within you for the entire time that you are pulling your hands toward your chest.

(3) When your hands reach your chest, exhale all of your breath in an explosive breath through the mouth. Take one deep inhale and exhale as you relax totally. Then repeat the exercise a few more times.

COOLING BREATH

The Cooling Breath is helpful in soothing the mind and releasing emotions such as anger, frustration, and anxiety. It also relaxes the muscles, brings the mind to a state of tranquility, and is great to practice before going to sleep since it generates a feeling of contentment.

Sit in Easy pose (p.19), with a straight spine. Straighten the arms and rest the hands in Gyan Mudra (p.21). Open your mouth and extend the tongue out. Curl the sides of the tongue upward and inhale through the mouth. The breath will produce a sound like rushing wind. Close the mouth and exhale through the nose. Continue this sequence for 3–11 minutes. If you cannot curl your tongue, shape your mouth like a circle and extend your tongue out while inhaling.

JAW RELEASE

This action relaxes and adjusts your jaw and helps improve jaw tension, which often results from stress-related habits such as clenching and grinding the teeth. It also releases tension around the ears and neck.

Lie down or sit in Easy pose (p.19). Begin to roll your tongue in a wide circle around the outside of your teeth while keeping your mouth closed. Move slowly, stretching your tongue as far as you can to reach every corner. Circle 5–8 times in one direction, then 5–8 times in the opposite direction.

HEALING POWER

Healing is as natural as breathing for a woman. Throughout the ages, we as women have healed through every aspect of ourselves. Through the compassionate touch of our hands, our poignant songs and art, the deep wisdom of our counsel, the conscious preparation of herbs and food, the life-giving milk that flows from our breasts, women's healing ways are infinitely creative and diverse. And through our deepest meditation, we become the empty cup—a space that our spirits fill to overflow. A woman in this state of consciousness heals with her presence. Her capacity to give is great, and she will often seek to heal others before herself. Yoga and meditation serve to restore her so that she can go on healing the world.

MOON SALUTATION

The connection between women and the Moon has always been strong. We resonate with the energy of the Moon through our monthly menstrual cycles, and reflect the Moon's pattern in the waxing and waning of our thoughts and feelings. For this reason, many women find that the practice of Moon Salutation holds special meaning for them. Practice 4–12 rounds of this strenuous sequence.

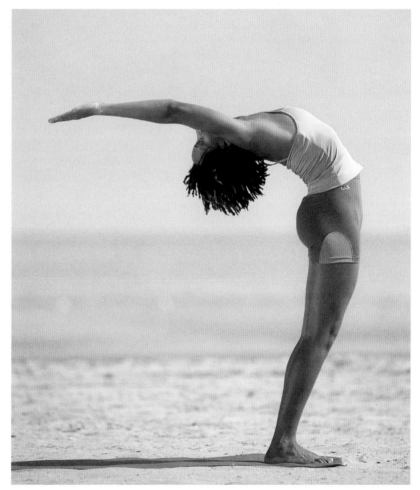

1. Stand upright with the feet close together. Bend the elbows and bring the palms of the hands together at the center of your chest. This centers the mind and calms the body.

2. Inhale slowly and deeply as you raise and stretch both arms above your head. At the same time, arch your upper body backward in one smooth, unbroken line, as far as possible without restraint. Bend only to your capacity, without strain. This stretches and tones the abdominal area, improves digestion, and opens the lungs, ready for step 3.

▶

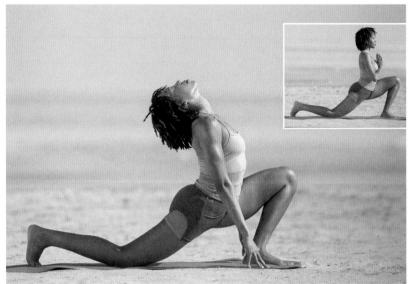

③ As you exhale slowly, bend forward until your fingers touch the ground on either side of the feet. Bring the head to the knees as far as possible without straining.

④ Inhale, stretch your right leg back as far as possible, and drop your right knee to the ground as you bend your left knee. The weight of the body is supported on both hands, the left foot, and the toes of the right foot. Lift your chest, arch your back and head upward, and bring your inner gaze to the brow point. This stretches and strengthens the muscles and nerves of the legs. Maintaining your balance, exhale and bring your palms together in front of your chest (inset).

⑤ Inhale as you stretch both arms over your head, keeping the palms together. Arch your back and look up, raising your chin as high as possible while inhaling to form a gentle curve resembling a crescent moon. Hold the position briefly, then exhale as you lower your hands to your chest (inset).

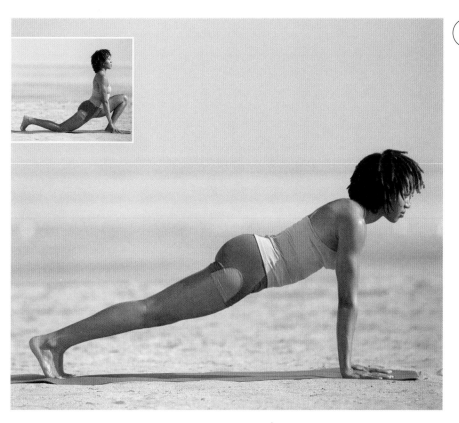

6 Inhale and return your hands to each side of your left foot (inset). Retaining the breath, bring your left leg back and place your left foot next to the right, toes pointing forward. Your arms are straight. Keep your head and hips in line with your spine. Your body should now be in a straight line, as in a push-up position.

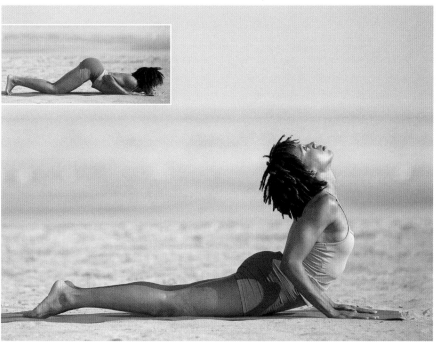

7 Exhale, lowering your knees, chest, and chin to the floor (inset). If this is not possible, first lower the knees, then the chest, and finally the chin. Inhale as you slide your body forward until the hips are on the ground. Arch your chest up and bring your head back into Cobra. Keep your elbows slightly bent as you curl back.

▶

(8) Keeping your hands and feet where they are, exhale and come onto the soles of your feet, lifting your hips into Downward Dog by pushing them up and back, away from your hands. Push your heels toward the ground and keep your knees straight. Stretch your spine and move your head inward, toward your feet.

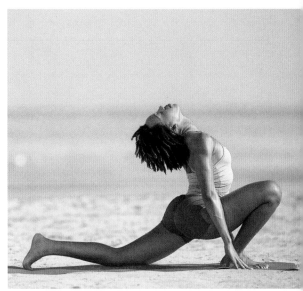

(9) Inhale and change legs, bringing your right foot forward between your hands. Drop your left knee toward the ground and stretch your head up. If, when you bring your foot forward, it does not align with your hands, slide your hands toward your body so that they frame the foot.

(10) Maintaining your balance, exhale and bring the palms together in front of your chest. Then stretch both arms over your head, keeping the palms together. Arch your back and look up, raising your chin as high as possible while inhaling.

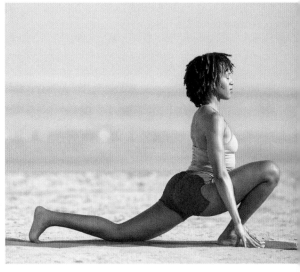

(11) Exhale as you lower your hands to your chest, then inhale once again and return your hands to each side of your right foot.

(12) Exhale slowly as you bring your left foot forward, straighten your legs, and stand up. Then bring your head down toward your knees.

(13) Inhale as you slowly bring your arms up over your head and stretch back. Tip the head back only as far as is comfortable.

(14) Exhale as you stand upright with your palms together at the center of your chest in the starting position. Repeat the sequence or end the set.

HEALING MEDITATION

The healing mantra *Ra Ma Da Sa, Sa Say So Hung* (the "a" in the first part of the mantra sounds like mama) translates as "Sun, Moon, Earth, Infinity—That I Am."

To practice, sit in Easy pose with a straight spine. Place a firm pillow under your buttocks if necessary. Bend the elbows and draw them into the sides of the rib cage. The palms of the hands face upward and are as flat as possible, creating a pressure at the wrists, and tipped at a 45° angle outward to the sides. Close your eyes and focus

between the eyebrows. Repeat the mantra once on each breath. Feel the navel pull slightly on the first *Sa* and on *Hung*. This is a strongly voiced, powerful chant that uses all the breath for each repetition. (For a musical version of this mantra, see the Music Resources on p.224.)

Continue the meditation for between 5 and 30 minutes. Then inhale, hold the breath, and focus your healing energy toward the person(s) that you are concentrating on for healing. Then relax quietly for a minute.

ENERGY FOR LIFE

When you have energy, you feel good and life
looks good. Positivity is effortless. When you feel
drained, it's a different story. Short tempers and
emotional outbursts abound. Or you switch over
to automatic pilot in a zombielike attempt just to
get through the day. Instead of reaching for a
candy bar or coffee, take a couple of minutes
to breathe and practice a few of the exercises
explained here. They can be practiced individually
or together to energize your body and brain. If
you have no more than a couple of minutes to
spare, try the quick-fix meditation on p.89,
making sure that you leave time to rest deeply
afterward. And in case you need a reminder,
you deserve to feel good!

BRIGHTEN UP

This fast-acting energizer can be done anytime you need a pick-me-up. It increases the flow of energy and oxygen to your brain and brightens your outlook. In the science of yoga, each area of the hand reflexes to a certain area of the body or brain. Your thumbs relate to your ego or unique personality. Stretching your thumbs upward activates a positive state of mind.

A regular yoga practice can benefit mental well-being. Brighten Up helps to oxygenate tissues and trigger the release of the mood-enhancing chemicals, dopamine and serotonin.

1 Sit between your heels, or alternatively on your heels. Lift your chest as you raise your arms to a 60° angle. Begin Breath of Fire. After 1–3 minutes, inhale deeply and hold the breath.

2 Slowly draw your thumbs together overhead on the held breath until the tips of your thumbs meet.

3 Exhale, opening the palms and slowly lowering your arms down in an arc around your body. As you lower your arms, imagine you are tracing the arc line of your aura—your surrounding field of energy.

SPRING BACK

Physically, this exercise works on revitalizing all the body systems and can be a great aerobic workout. Mentally, it gives you the ability to spring back into life. It gives you an edge because it helps you to think fast. A woman must be physically active in order to have this edge.

(1) Stand with your feet shoulder-width apart and knees slightly bent. Your hands are in fists, with the palms facing each other in front of the chest.

(2) As you exhale, punch forward with the left arm while simultaneously springing off the ground and bringing the left leg forward and the right leg back into a front stance position. During the jump, your right fist pulls back to the right side of your chest.

(3) Spring back to the original position (step 1) on your next inhalation. Continue this action on the same side for 1–2 minutes, then change sides. The jumping movement should be light and fast.

BUNDLE ROLL

The tightening of the body in Bundle Roll strengthens muscle mass, as well as strengthening your entire nervous system. It is good for relieving hyperactivity and anxiety in adults and children. Be sure to have soft padding underneath you as you practice Bundle Roll. Give yourself a whole-body massage!

① Lie down on your back with your arms straight at your sides (inset). Stiffen your body, point your toes, and begin to rock from side to side until you flip over to one side. Keep your body straight.

② Flip onto your front, then roll from front to back and back to front, flipping over and over without bending. Maintain tension in your entire body throughout. Continue for 2–3 minutes, then relax on your back or front for a minute.

BRIDGE

This pose massages and invigorates the digestive organs and is excellent for general strengthening of the ovaries and uterus. Bridge is a good preparation for Wheel (p.90) or can be practiced as an alternative to it.

A strong pose, Bridge stimulates blood flow to the reproductive organs in the pelvic region, nourishing and oxygenating the tissues to help optimize reproductive health.

① Lie on your back with your knees bent. Place the feet flat on the ground close to the buttocks. Reach down and grasp each ankle with the respective hands, or place your hands on the ground beside you with the palms down.

② Keeping the feet, head, and upper shoulders on the ground, roll up. Start with your pelvis and follow with your upper spine. Lift as high as is comfortable as you inhale, then roll down as you exhale. As you roll down, lead with your upper spine and follow with the lower. Continue this sequence for 1–2 minutes, then stretch up once more and begin Breath of Fire (p.24) for 1 minute before rolling back down.

Rolling up and down enhances the elasticity of the spine and massages all the back muscles

MEDITATION FOR ABSOLUTELY POWERFUL ENERGY

Only 2 minutes are needed to relieve "brain drain," or mental fatigue, with this meditation. It is important to allow resting time afterward.

1 Sit in Easy pose with a straight spine. Place your palms together. Keep your ring fingers together and extended as you interlace and fold down the other fingers (inset).

2 Hold your hands several inches out from your solar plexus/diaphragm area. Your extended fingers point up at a 60° angle.

3 Close your eyes. Inhale deeply through the nose but keep your mouth open. Chant the mantra *Ong*

(p.22), extending the sound through your nasal passages as "Ooonnnnng." Sense the sound coming from the upper back area of your soft palate at the juncture of the throat and nasal passages. As you chant, your navel will pull back slightly toward your spine and your attention will naturally flow upward to the sixth chakra (your brow point). Repeat five times, or continue for longer if you wish. Then rest or go to sleep.

COUNTERPOSE FOR BRIDGE AND WHEEL

Tuck your knees into your chest with your hands on your shins and breathe deeply for 20 seconds to 1 minute.

WHEEL

Besides the Wheel's obvious benefits of increasing the flexibility of the spine and strengthening the muscles of the abdomen, legs, and arms, this powerful pose energizes your mental faculties; improves your memory; and is extremely beneficial for your glandular system, especially the lymph system. Inverted postures such as Wheel, Shoulderstand (pp.52–53), and Plow (pp.114–115) literally and figuratively "turn you upside down," giving you a new perspective on life.

Preparing for wheel

1 Lift up as high as possible in Bridge (p.88), then bring your hands to the ground behind the shoulders. The palms should be flat on the ground with the fingers pointing toward the shoulders.

2 Arch your body farther upward as your arms and feet press into the ground. Your neck will arch back as you bring the top of your head to the ground. Take a few deep breaths, then relax down slowly, releasing your neck carefully. Stay at this level as long as you like before trying the full pose.

Full wheel

① Lie on your back with your knees bent. Place the feet flat on the ground close to the buttocks. Bring your hands to the ground behind your shoulders, palms flat on the ground with the fingers pointing toward the shoulders.

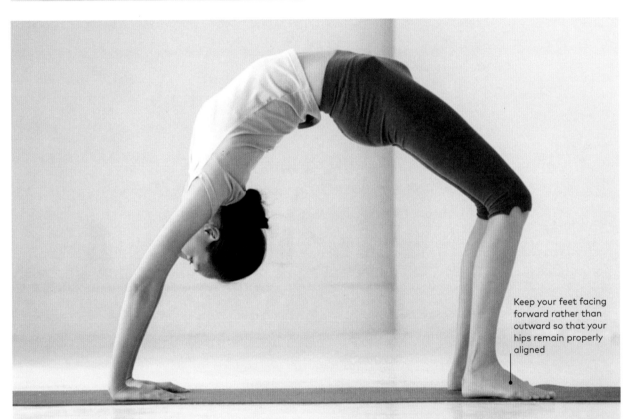

Keep your feet facing forward rather than outward so that your hips remain properly aligned

② Inhale and lift your body upward, straightening your elbows and arching your hips and chest up as high as possible. Allow your head to drop back. Do deep breathing or Breath of Fire (p.24) for between 30 seconds and 2 minutes.

③ Come down carefully and gently from the pose, starting with the upper body, and rest in counterpose (p.89).

LIGHTENING UP

How do we develop the power to love ourselves as we are and to change the things that we find no longer serve us? In yoga, often the answer is "navel power." In Lightening Up, we'll work directly with this power source—the navel center, third chakra energy. In the womb, the navel was your original source of power through the nourishment you received from your mother. Now the navel center is the seat of your physical well-being and your ability to hold your intention and make it manifest. Here, you'll recharge your navel batteries, so to speak. This creates an internal heat, called tapas, that is self-empowering. The activated power is drawn upward into the higher chakras with poses that lighten your heart and mind.

ALTERNATE LEG LIFTS

Leg raises aid the proper functioning of the intestines and create an internal energy that activates the navel area. Coupled with strong, deep breaths, they revitalize the abdominal area and strengthen the back and thighs.

(1) Lie on your back with your arms down at your sides, palms facing downward.

(2) Inhale and lift your right leg straight up to a 90° angle, then exhale and lower it. Repeat with the left leg. Keep the knee straight but not locked and lift from the hip. Continue raising and lowering alternate legs with deep and powerful breaths for 2–4 minutes.

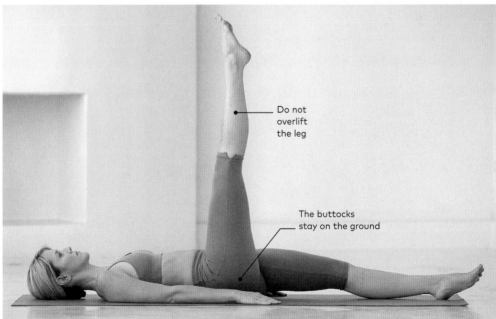

Do not overlift the leg

The buttocks stay on the ground

TREE POSE

This balancing pose adjusts the vertebrae of the spine and promotes good posture. It refreshes and uplifts the mind. Beginners may want to practice standing with one shoulder next to a wall for support.

1 Stand tall on a firm surface with your feet close together and your arms at your sides.

2 Place your left foot inside your right thigh. Ideally, it will rest close to the top of the inner thigh, but it can be placed toward the inside of the knee.

3 Steady yourself in this pose by focusing the eyes straight ahead. Breathe deeply and bring the palms together at the heart center.

Focus on the upward stretch through the spine, rib cage, neck, and arms

After years of struggling with the female inclination to obsess over body image and food issues, I have come to some understandings about myself: the happier I am, the less I judge myself, inside or out; and the happier I am, the more I feel like eating well and in moderation. So being happy is the key. What I've also discovered is that no one makes me happy—I make myself happy. The ball is in my court and in my hands at all times. Happiness for me equals being at peace with myself.

4 When you feel ready, slowly inhale and stretch the palms up toward the sky, straightening the arms so that they are close to the sides of the head. Keep the spine straight and feel your whole body lift upward. Continue in Tree pose for 1–3 minutes, then come out of the pose slowly and switch sides.

LIFT AND LAUGH

The angle of the first part of this exercise moves the activated navel energy into the heart and upper centers of the body. Belly laughing is good for the soul. It also stokes the fires of digestion.

1 Sit with your legs stretched out together in front of you and place your hands behind you so that your body is positioned at a 45° angle to the ground.

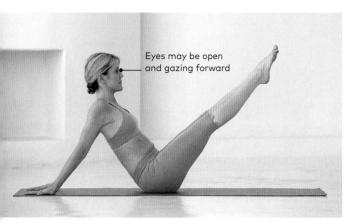

Eyes may be open and gazing forward

2 Point your toes and lean back slightly, keeping the back straight and the chest lifted. Lift your legs to a 60° angle and hold with Breath of Fire (p.24) for 1–2 minutes. Then inhale deeply, exhale, and hold the out breath. Apply Root Lock (p.25). Then relax the breath, the lock, and the posture.

3 Immediately sit in Easy pose (p.19) and begin belly laughing. Use your navel and laugh loudly! Enjoy the ridiculousness of doing this.

SA TA NA MA MEDITATION

Sa Ta Na Ma is one of the most well-practiced meditations in the Kundalini tradition. It is a clearing house for unwanted thoughts and feelings and is especially effective as part of your morning yoga practice or before bed for a restful sleep (see also Music Resources, p.224).

Sit in Easy pose with a straight spine, your hands on your knees. Your thumbs sequentially press each finger as you chant the mantra: *Sa* (Totality), press the thumb and index finger; *Ta* (Creation), press the thumb and middle finger; *Na* (Dissolution), press the thumb and ring finger; *Ma* (Regeneration), press the thumb and little finger. Continue pressing the fingers sequentially and chanting out loud for 2 minutes. This is the voice of the human. Continue the finger movements, whispering for 2 minutes. This is the voice of the beloved. Next chant silently, hearing the mantra internally while still moving the fingers for 2 minutes. This is the inner voice. Reverse the process: 2 minutes of silent repetition,

2 minutes of whispering, and 2 minutes of chanting out loud. Work up to 5 minutes for each part of the meditation. As you repeat the mantra, imagine the sound of each syllable entering through the crown center and leaving through the sixth center between the eyebrows. This energy flow strengthens the connection in the brain, clearing the subconscious mind and allowing access to the higher centers of the brain. Pressing the fingertips activates meridian points in the hands that also help energy flow to the brain centers.

Dr. Dharma Singh Khalsa presents an experiment in his book, *Meditation as Medicine*, in which a PET scan was done on a practitioner of this meditation. Different areas of the brain lit up as the fingers were pressed, showing that the various finger movements have a direct impact on brain function. One study found that brief daily meditation practices can lead to improved mental and cognitive functioning and lower levels of depressive symptoms.

Sa: thumb, index finger

Ta: thumb, middle finger

Na: thumb, ring finger

Ma: thumb, little finger

BALANCING

From her youth up to the "wise woman" status of her middle years, a woman's menstrual cycle profoundly affects her life. This one feature makes all the difference on every level—mental, physical, and emotional. Each stage of life—from the onset of menstruation to menopause— holds challenges and gifts.

Balance is the key to turning these challenges into gifts. In practicing specific yoga exercises for dealing with PMS, mood swings, and menopausal symptoms, a balance comes into your life—a sense of well-being. No matter what your current phase of life, these chapters have something priceless to offer—an opportunity to experience calm in the midst of the storm.

LEVELING OUT

Whether it's because of fluctuating hormones
or a refined sensitivity we are born with, emotions
play a key role in women's lives. We may
overreact, take things too hard, project our own
pain into situations, or just get out of balance.
But what can seem like a curse can also be seen
as a blessing. We are blessed to be aware,
sensitive beings. Whether the issue is depression,
manic behavior, or both alternately, the first
step in evening out highs and lows is to pick up
one foot and put it down. Then continue to place
one foot in front of the other until you are
standing on your yoga mat. Promptly sit down,
tune in, and get ready to feel better with
yoga and meditation for balance,
clarity, and stability.

BALANCING POSES

The intricate connection between body, mind, and spirit is quite apparent in the practice of balancing poses. Working with these poses strengthens your focus and brings your mind to a neutral place. The more focused and stable you are, the easier it is to remain steady in your practice.

TRIANGLE

This pose stretches the spine and spinal nerves laterally, helps to adjust the sacrum and lower back, and stretches the muscles and nerves in the legs and arms. It reduces stress and anxiety through its capacity to center and balance you.

① Stand with the feet 3–4 ft (1–1.2 m) apart and your arms raised so that they are straight out to the sides at shoulder level.

② Pivot your right foot 90° to the right and turn your left foot in slightly by moving the heel outward. Check your right heel is in line with the arch of your left foot and that the weight is evenly distributed. Keep your pelvis facing forward and your shoulders relaxed, broaden from the center of your chest, and breathe deeply a few times before continuing on with step 3. ▶

(3) Inhale, lower your right arm, and bring it to rest on your shin. Extend your left arm up from the shoulder with the palm facing forward. Exhale and shift your pelvis to the left while moving the shoulders toward the right, bringing the right shoulder out and over the right leg. Keep your chest and pelvis open and facing forward. Take a few deep breaths.

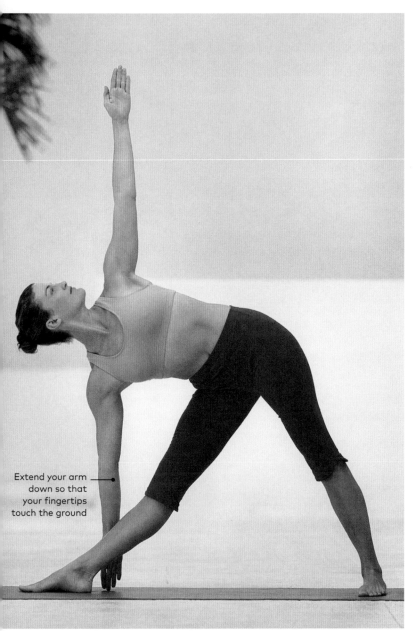

Extend your arm down so that your fingertips touch the ground

④ Slide the hand down toward the ankle, as far as you can without rotating the left hip forward. Fully extend both arms, keeping them in alignment with each other and straight out from the shoulders. Look up toward the extended arm, straight ahead, or down at your foot. Relax and breathe as you hold the position for 30 seconds to 1 minute.

⑤ To come out of the pose, exhale, press through the ball of your left foot, and lift, keeping the spine elongated. If you feel unsteady, bend the left knee to lift out of the pose. Then turn your feet to face forward, as in step 1; take a few breaths; and practice Triangle pose on the other side with the left leg extended.

CROW

This pose strengthens the arms, wrists, and shoulders and lubricates the joints, tendons, and ligaments of the upper body. The intense focus on balance strengthens the nervous system and provides excellent powers of concentration. Crow also encourages a feeling of inner balance and prepares the mind for meditation.

If you are new to Crow, put a folded blanket or firm pillow in front of your hands in case you tumble forward.

(1) Come into a squatting position, with the feet flat on the ground and the arms between the knees. Place your palms flat on the ground and spread your fingers far apart and turned slightly inward, like the feet of a crow.

(2) Bend your elbows outward so that your upper arms can act as a support for your knees. Rise up onto the balls of your feet and rest your knees on each upper arm.

(3) Keep your head facing forward, with your eyes focused on a point a little way in front of you. Inhale deeply. Hold the breath as you gradually shift your weight forward onto your hands so that your toes hardly touch the ground. Stay at this level until you can balance comfortably, or experiment by carefully lifting your toes off the ground for a few seconds at a time.

(4) Keep your head up by focusing out in front of you and shift the balance of weight entirely onto the hands, slowly lifting the feet off the floor. If this proves difficult, try raising one foot and then the other. Ideally, your knees are resting on the upper arms and the lower legs are parallel to the ground with the feet relaxed. Breathe deeply and hold for as long as is comfortable.

YOGA FOR MENTAL AND EMOTIONAL BALANCE

This yoga set balances the pelvis and adjusts the navel area, which opens up nerve channels and builds pranic life energy. Strong backbends and dynamic arm movements then encourage the pranic energy to flow through to higher chakras, activating the heart center and bringing the mind into a state of equipoise.

1 MIRACLE BEND

This pose activates the navel center, which in turn helps to give a woman the ability to find her inner security, balance her emotions, and let go of depression. It also helps to process strong emotions and, if practiced with deep breathing, it can bring about a sense of calm.

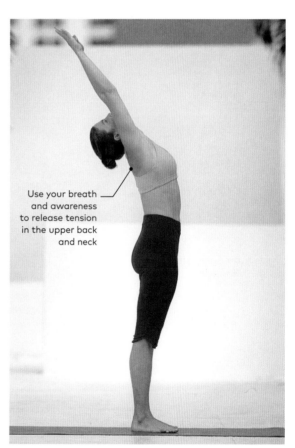

Use your breath and awareness to release tension in the upper back and neck

① Stand with your heels together and your toes angled outward for balance. Bring your arms straight out in front of you, with the hands close together and the fingers straightened. The thumbs may be crossed over each other.

② Begin to inhale deeply as you raise your extended arms upward and backward in a smooth, flowing motion. Your head and upper body follow your arms so that your arms, head, and upper body form an unbroken curve, lifted upward and backward as far as possible. Breathe deeply and slowly as you hold the position for 1–2 minutes.

▶

Move as if in
slow motion

Take 30–45
seconds to come
fully forward

3 Exhale deeply and slowly begin to straighten your body and smoothly bend it forward to
   your maximum capacity. Keep your arms and head moving together in an unbroken line.
   Then inhale, retain the breath within the rib cage, and for as long as possible begin to
   pump your navel, pressing it in toward your spine and releasing. Continue until you have
   to exhale, then do the same on the held exhalation. Inhale and continue this pumping
   pattern on the held inhalation and exhalation for 2 minutes.

4 Come out of the pose by rolling upward
   gradually while inhaling slowly and
   deeply. Uncurl one vertebra at a time
   in a slow, fluid motion.

2 HIP CIRCLES

Hip circles bring flexibility to the pelvis since the lower spine and hips are adjusted and balanced in this movement. Mentally, this exercise gives you the spirit to keep going and to not give in.

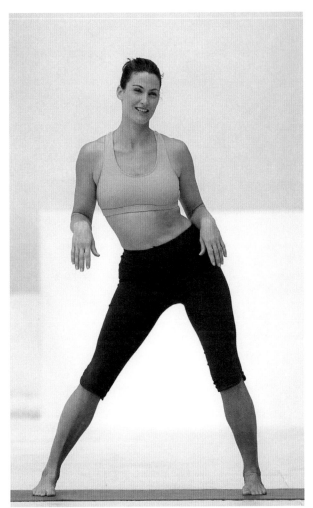

① Stand tall, placing your feet far apart while maintaining your balance. Distribute your weight evenly across the soles of your feet. Keep your knees straight but not locked. Bring your elbows toward your sides and bend them so that your forearms are more or less parallel to the ground and your hands are relaxed.

② Begin to rotate your hips in large circles in one direction. Widen the circles as you continue for 1 minute. Breathe deeply as you circle. Then reverse the direction and repeat the movement for 1 minute more.

3 ALTERNATE ARM CIRCLES

This exercise helps with stamina, clear thinking, and balance during menopause. Though there is no breathing pattern specified, you may want to inhale as you bend in one direction and exhale on the other.

This active sequence is centering and energizing. It brings balance to body and mind and builds stamina to help deal with the fatigue that can sometimes accompany menopause.

(1) Stand with your feet 3–4 ft (1–1.2 m) apart. Straighten your arms and begin rotating them in backward circles, starting with one arm and then bringing in the other arm, so that the arms circle alternately. Your arms are positioned out to the sides, away from the body, throughout.

(2) Bend the torso forward from the waist while continuing to move the arms in alternate circles. When you have bent forward halfway, begin to straighten up again as you circle.

(3) Without breaking the movement, bend backward halfway, or as far as possible. The rhythm is around 15 seconds for a complete cycle of forward and backward bends. Keep circling the arms the entire time as you continue for 1–2 minutes.

MEDITATION TO DEAL WITH LIFE

This meditation totally recharges you and is an antidote to depression. It gives you the capacity and caliber to deal with life as it is. It strengthens your pranic life energy—your internal energy system for making optimum use of the vital life force of the breath. When the prana flows through the nadis, or energy pathways, the cells of the body come alive with vitality and toxins are released.

Sit in Easy pose (p.19) with a straight spine. Extend your arms out straight in front of you, slightly below shoulder level and parallel to the ground. Close your right hand into a fist. Wrap your left hand around the right so that the fingers of the left hand are over the knuckles of the right fist. The heels of the hands touch each other. Straighten the thumbs, extending them up so that the sides are touching. Focus your eyes so that you gaze at your thumbs. Inhale for 5 seconds, then exhale for 5 seconds. Exhale completely and hold the breath out for 15 seconds. Then inhale and continue the pattern. Do not retain the inhalation; suspend the breath out of the body on the exhale only.

Start with 3–5 minutes of this powerful breathing meditation, then build the time gradually to 11 minutes. Eventually you can work up to holding the breath out longer, up to a maximum of 1 minute, but always increase the time slowly and moderately according to your natural capability.

Wrap fingers around fist

Thumbs should touch

MONTHLY CYCLE

Throughout history, women have viewed the menstrual cycle as everything from an annoyance to "The Curse." In some indigenous cultures, however, this special time is referred to as a woman's "moon cycle." Once a month, a woman will set aside her usual roles of caregiver, counselor, and innovator to enter a phase of self-nurturing retreat and inner communion with the divine feminine for the duration of her menstrual cycle.

Here, you will have the same opportunity for meditative retreat using specially selected yoga exercises. You will also find yoga that strengthens your reproductive health so that you may enjoy being a woman in every way.

DURING A CYCLE

As we shed the old during menstruation and prepare for a new monthly cycle, we feel the instinct to let go to make room for the new. Folding the body forward is a natural gesture of letting go and is usually accompanied by deep, extended exhalations. Allow the natural force of gravity to help you relax forward in these poses especially for the menstrual cycle.

Forward bends such as Folded Butterfly stimulate blood flow to the ovaries, nourishing this area. As the body comes forward, the lower back muscles are also stretched and warmed, helping to relieve the heavy feeling that can occur here during menstruation.

FOLDED BUTTERFLY

This pose stretches and strengthens the lower back and hip areas. The forward stretch at the end soothes the ovaries and abdomen and helps to relieve lower back pain during menstruation.

1 Sitting in Easy pose, bring the soles of the feet together in front of you, as close to your body as is comfortable.

2 Hold onto your feet and flap your knees for 30 seconds to relax your hips.

3 With your hands on your feet, gently bring your head toward your feet and hold the posture. This may be easier if you move your feet a few more inches away from your body. Breathe long and deep for 1 minute, sending the inhalation to your hips, lower spine, and reproductive organs for healing and relaxation. Then exhale any remaining tension from those areas.

EXTENDED CHILD'S POSE

Extended Child's pose relieves tension from the ovaries and revitalizes the glandular system, so it is excellent during the premenstrual period, as well as during menstruation. Practicing regular Child's pose is also excellent for releasing abdominal and reproductive tension.

Bringing the body down to the ground has a profoundly restful and calming effect on the body and mind, relieving stress and anxiety and promoting an inner calm.

(1) Sit on your heels in Rock pose (p.20) with your spine straight.

Refrain from cold showers, Body Locks, inverted poses (such as Shoulderstand), abdominal poses (such as Stretch pose), and backbends (such as Bow) during a period. Do only light Breath of Fire.

(2) Place your hands on the ground in front of your knees. Shift your weight forward onto your hands. Extend one leg straight out behind you, with the top of the foot resting on the ground.

Allow your shoulders to drop forward

(3) Bring your forehead to the ground and relax your arms by your sides with your palms facing up. Allow your entire body to relax. Your hands will naturally curl slightly. Allow your shoulders to drop forward. Feel your hips and buttocks relax and spread, and drop all tension from your straightened leg. Take long, deep breaths for 1–3 minutes, then switch legs by supporting your body with your forearms as you sit up slowly and come back to position 1.

REPRODUCTIVE HEALTH

The following two poses build reproductive and glandular health. Although they may not be comfortable to practice during menstruation, they can be practiced all other times of the month, either together or individually.

PLOW

Plow is said to benefit the entire body, especially the throat, thyroid, and circulation. The muscles of the back, shoulders, and arms are stretched and strengthened. Plow also provides an inverted gravitational pull that suspends and relaxes all your internal organs, including your reproductive organs. After Plow, be sure to rest on your back for a minute or two with the legs out straight or with a firm pillow under the knees. If your feet do not easily reach the ground in Plow, position yourself so that they rest against a wall. To relieve pressure from the neck, use a prop (p.52).

Ginger tea

At once calming to the nerves and energizing to the body and mind, ginger tea is good at any time and is especially helpful for women during their monthly menses.

Boil 4–6 thin slices of fresh ginger root (unpeeled is fine) in 2 cups of water. Boil for about 20 minutes until the water is light brown in color. Add a bit of fresh lemon juice and honey to taste.

① Lie on your back, your arms at your sides and palms facing downward. Using your abdominal muscles and the pressure of your arms against the floor, raise your legs and buttocks up.

Move your hands farther up your back to stretch more deeply

② Lift your buttocks and lower back off the ground while supporting your back with your hands, which are positioned at the waist. Rest your elbows firmly on the floor. Bring your legs overhead as you come up onto your upper back and shoulders. Your chin will be close to your chest.

CHEEK PRESS

Using your thumbs, find the indentations directly under your cheekbones. Press strongly and hold in each position for three breaths. This releases facial tension. For a deeper release of tension, begin to press all along that ridge, massaging the muscle under the cheekbones from the inside area close to your nose to the outer edge where it meets your jaw.

3 Straighten your legs and, if possible without straining, bring your feet to the ground behind your head. Once you feel stable in this position, bring your hands to the ground beside you with your palms facing downward. Relax and breathe for 1–3 minutes.

With your toes on the floor, gently push the heels toward the ground

4 Roll out of this position slowly by exhaling and rolling your spine down, vertebra by vertebra, using your hands on the ground for support.

The functioning of the thyroid gland is susceptible to the depleting effects of chronic stress. Plow inverts the body and concentrates blood flow to the throat, stimulating the thyroid and encouraging efficient circulation.

COBRA

This pose increases flexibility and rejuvenates the spinal nerves. Combined with deep breathing or Breath of Fire (p.24), it massages and expands the rib cage. Cobra is particularly helpful for relieving tension in the ovaries and uterus, often the cause of menstrual problems. Cobra stimulates the flow of pranic energy in the body and awakens the higher chakras.

Rolling the pelvic area and abdomen off the ground in Cobra gives the ovaries and uterus an internal massage, toning and warming these areas to soothe menstrual discomfort.

① Lie down on your front with your arms resting at your sides and your chin on the ground. Take a deep breath.

② Keeping your lower body relaxed, place your hands on the ground under your shoulders to prepare for Cobra.

③ Lead with the head and chest and curve your spine up and back into Cobra as you inhale. Exhale and relax more deeply into Cobra. Continue holding the posture for 1–3 minutes with deep breathing or Breath of Fire. Then inhale deeply, exhale, and slowly lower the chest, then the head, down. Rest for a few breaths with your arms at your sides and your head turned to one side.

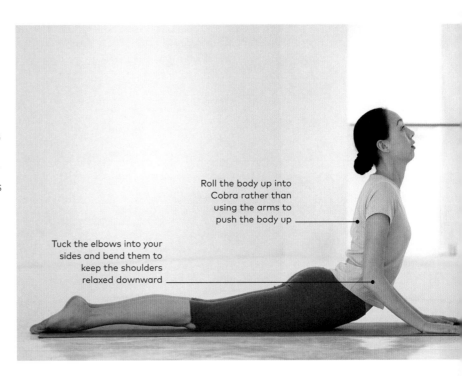

Roll the body up into Cobra rather than using the arms to push the body up

Tuck the elbows into your sides and bend them to keep the shoulders relaxed downward

MEDITATION TO BALANCE THE MENSTRUAL CYCLE

An erratic menstrual cycle can be regulated through a steady practice of this meditation. Negative thought patterns are released and in their place comes mental clarity, positivity, and a radiant aura. This breath meditation uses the "broken breath" technique. The inhalation is broken into four equal sections, while the exhalation is one long breath. In yogic teachings, this type of breathing pattern is used to heal oneself and break depression.

On a physical level, the positive attitude of this four-part breathing meditation rejuvenates the pituitary and pineal glands, which are crucial for the emotional and physical health and well-being of the whole person. All other body systems rely on the "ductless glands" of the endocrine system since they regulate the hormones that keep you fit, healthy, and mentally stable.

1 Sit in Easy pose with your hands resting on your knees, palms facing upward. You will be breaking the inhalation into four equal parts. Each part will be a short "sniff," and you will feel your navel press slightly inward on each of the sniffs if you are practicing it correctly. On each sniff, press your thumb and one of your fingers as follows:

On the first sniff, press your thumb and first finger as you meditate on the sound *Sa*.

On the second, press your thumb and second finger as you meditate on the sound *Ta*.

On the third, press your thumb and third finger as you meditate on the sound *Na*.

And on the fourth and final sniff, press your thumb and little finger as you meditate on the sound *Ma*.

2 Exhale in one long stroke. Continue with the four-part inhalation, meditating on *Sa Ta Na Ma*, for 3 minutes.

The length of time for this meditation may be increased by 1 minute daily, up to 7 minutes, then practice for a week or more at 7 minutes. After that, increase the meditation again by a minute per day. The maximum time for this powerful meditation is 31 minutes.

For a complete explanation of the *Sa Ta Na Ma* meditation, see p.97.

EASING INTO MENOPAUSE

With the right combination of attitude and holistic lifestyle—a healthy plant-based diet, daily yoga and meditation, and supplements and herbs (as well as hormone replacement therapy if needed)—menopause can be, dare I say it, a blessing! Hearing these words, those of you who are going through nightmarish symptoms of hot flashes, long nights of erratic sleep, and irritability bordering on rage can comfort yourselves that you may be heading toward that point at this very moment!

Every woman's experience is unique; there are as many different stories about menopause as there are women. Encouragingly, a Gallup survey showed that more than half of American women between the ages of 50 and 65 felt happiest and most fulfilled at this stage of life.

I believe that once the physical and emotional challenges become manageable, many women make a miraculous discovery about menopause—that it heralds a new consciousness; a new way of looking at life; and even, if one is brave and bold, a new life itself. Menopause gives us cause to stop in our well-worn tracks and ask, "What am I all about? What do I really want? What calls to me?"

Dr. Christiane Northrup draws upon her own personal experience in her book, *The Wisdom of Menopause*, which reveals the difficult and liberating process of the life change that is initiated through menopause. These changes can be wonderfully life-affirming, a time of personal empowerment and positive energy. As Dr. Northrup writes: *"Our brains are changing. A woman's thoughts, her ability to focus, and the amount of fuel going to the intuitive centers in the temporal lobes of her brain all are plugged into, and affected by, the circuits being rewired. After working with thousands of women who are going through this process, as well as experiencing it myself, I can say with great assurance that menopause is an exciting developmental stage—one that, when participated in consciously, holds enormous promise for transforming and healing our bodies, minds, and spirits at the deepest levels."*

Body, mind, and spirit is what yoga is all about. Although all yoga postures and exercises are helpful for smoothing out the rough edges of menopause, here the spotlight will focus particularly on hormonal balance, supporting the nervous system, and our reproductive health and will end with a meditation to balance the emotions and bring the mind to a state of equipoise and elevation.

SUPPORT FOR GOOD MENOPAUSAL HEALTH

This group of poses can help to reduce many of the most common symptoms of menopause, such as hot flashes, mood swings, undue weight gain, or sleeplessness. They particularly rejuvenate the reproductive organs and stimulate the proper working of the glandular system. They can each be practiced with either deep breathing or Breath of Fire. Feel free to practice them together or individually.

Fish pose revitalizes the abdominal organs and the digestive system, improving their efficiency. Blood flow to the pelvic area is also increased, promoting reproductive health.

FISH POSE

This pose opens the hips and pelvis and revitalizes the entire digestive and reproductive areas. If needed, place several folded blankets or a firm pillow or bolster behind your back before lying down. Be sure to support your neck with a rolled towel or small pillow.

① Sit between or on your heels. If your heels feel overpressured, place a rolled towel or pillow between your thighs and calves.

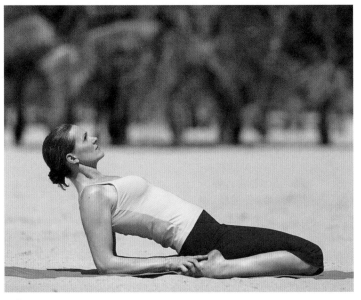

② Bring your elbows down to the ground behind you, lean back, and ease yourself into a lying position, with your hands grasping the soles of your feet. Take care not to strain the neck.

Easy-does-it version
Begin in Easy pose (p.19). Supporting your body with your elbows on the ground, lean back until you are lying down on your back with your legs still crossed in Easy pose.

③ Once you are lying down, relax your shoulders and expand your chest and hips with each breath. Relax your arms by your sides, palms facing upward. Hold for 1–2 minutes.

④ To come out of the pose, use your abdominal and upper body muscles to gently bring yourself back up onto your elbows and then to an upright sitting position. Take care to keep the neck relaxed throughout.

⑤ Sit up straight and release your legs. Then stretch your legs out and enjoy a Forward Hang (p.73) for a few seconds.

DOWNWARD FACING DOG

With regular practice, Downward Facing Dog rejuvenates your whole body. An inverted pose, it allows for the reversed flow of gravity and increases the flow of blood to the head and heart. It reduces stiffness in the shoulders, legs, and heels and makes the legs strong and agile for walking and running. If practiced regularly, it can help halt heavy menstrual flow and help prevent hot flashes during menopause. If you have low blood pressure, come out of the position gradually to avoid dizziness. This pose is easier to do on a yoga mat.

Beginners may use a bolster to support the head. To facilitate this pose without strain to the legs and feet, use a prop such as a block of wood under each hand to shorten the distance between the hands and the feet.

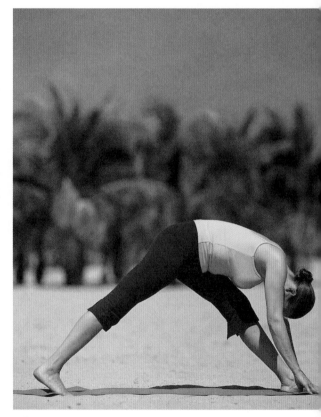

① Stand up straight at the front edge of your mat, your arms at your sides.

② Exhale and bend over at the waist, placing your hands on the ground beside your feet. If your hands do not reach the ground easily, bend your knees.

③ As you inhale, step back with one foot so that your foot is approximately 3–4 ft (1–1.2 m) away from your hands. Step back with the other foot so that it aligns with the first foot. Both hands and feet are now about 3–4 ft (1–1.2 m) apart.

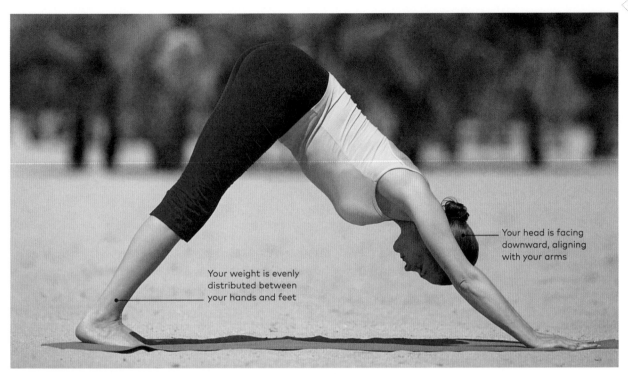

Your head is facing downward, aligning with your arms

Your weight is evenly distributed between your hands and feet

4 Position your right leg so that it is in line with your right arm and your left leg is in line with your left arm. Stretch and open your fingers and toes. Feel the stretch from your palms to your heels. Move your torso toward your legs. Keep your hips lifted and stretched upward and backward. If possible, stretch your heels down to the ground. Slightly lower the crown of your head toward the ground. Continue stretching in this position for 1–2 minutes.

5 To come out of the pose, inhale as you bend one knee and step forward, bringing the foot as close to the hands as possible. Continue to support yourself with your hands on the ground.

6 Step the other leg forward while exhaling, bringing both feet into alignment. Bend your knees slightly if necessary. Then inhale and stand up straight. You may like to repeat the pose on the other leg.

CHAIR

This is an excellent pose for bringing energy and improved blood circulation to the ovaries, uterus, and pelvic area. It strengthens the leg muscles and opens the hips. It also helps activate the energy of the first three chakras (p.15) and circulates that energy into the solar plexus (emotional balance) and heart (compassion, selfless service) chakras. If your heels do not reach the floor comfortably, roll or fold a towel or blanket to place under your heels while in this position.

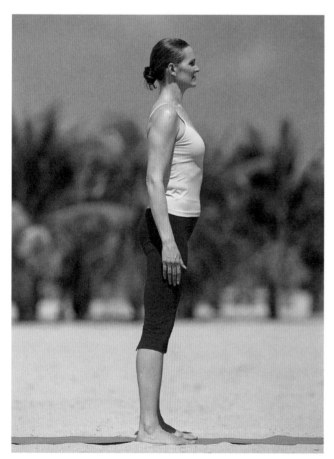

① Stand up straight with your feet about 24 in (60 cm) apart, parallel to each other and facing forward. Inhale deeply.

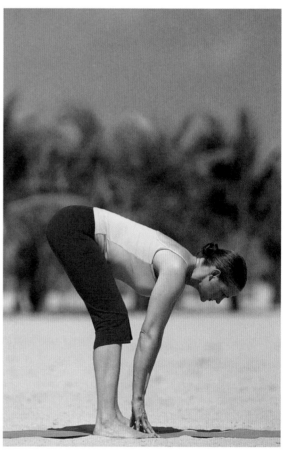

② Exhale as you bend forward, keeping the back straight and your head facing forward. Bend your knees so that your hands reach the floor. Your arms will be close to the inside of your bent knees.

3 Inhale, then exhale and lean forward slightly while bringing your hands between your legs. Turn your palms to face your ankles and grasp your heels (or ankles if necessary). Keep your head, spine, and buttocks in alignment and parallel to the floor. Breathe normally for 1–2 minutes.

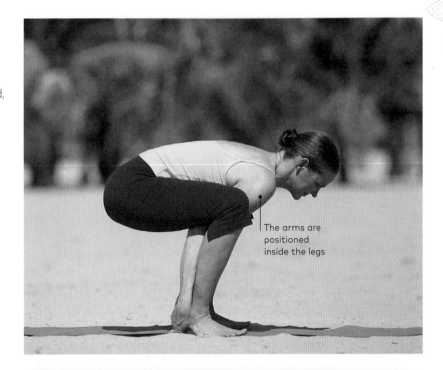

The arms are positioned inside the legs

4 To come out of Chair pose, place your hands on the ground in front of your feet and push up, straightening your legs. Relax in a Forward Hang (p.73) with the legs straight for a few seconds as you exhale.

PIGEON

Pigeon pose increases flexibility in the hips and groin and stretches the thigh muscles. It expands the chest, strengthens the lungs, and facilitates deep breathing. This pose strengthens the back muscles and revitalizes the kidneys and the entire endocrine system.

A healthy endocrine system (adrenals, reproductive glands, pancreas, thyroid) means a well-integrated connection between mind, body, and emotions.

① Begin by sitting on your heels and bringing your forearms to the ground with the palms facing downward.

② Slide your left knee forward between your elbows and your right leg straight out behind you. Square your hips to the front and lie the right foot flat on the ground. Lower your left hip toward the ground. If this is uncomfortable or feels unsteady, place a blanket under your left hip to support it. If needed, stay in this position or go on to step 3.

③ Draw your upper body upright and place your fingertips on the floor on either side of your bent knee. Relax your shoulders and lengthen your spine through the crown of your head as you inhale, lifting your sternum and pressing your heart center forward. Look straight ahead and breathe deeply for 1–2 minutes.

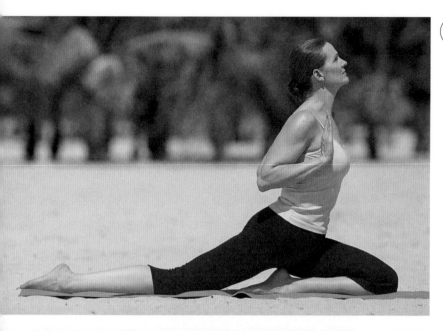

4 Practice this move when you feel you have gained enough flexibility and stability; otherwise, go on to step 5. Bring your arms up to shoulder level, with your elbows pressing into your sides and your palms facing forward. Let your eyes gaze up at the sky with your spine straight, chest lifted, and chin tipped slightly upward. Hold the position with deep breathing for 1–2 minutes.

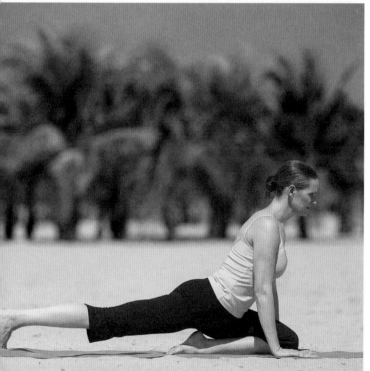

5 To come out of Pigeon, bring your hands down to either side of your front knee. Press your hands into the ground and lower your torso forward slightly as you lift your hips away from the ground.

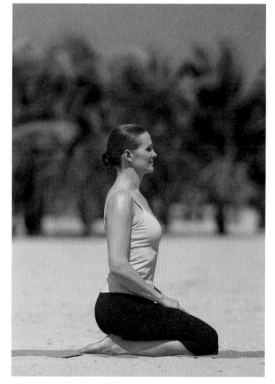

6 Bring your right knee forward so that you finish by sitting in Rock pose (p.20). Then repeat the pose with your left leg extended and your right leg bent.

FRONT LUNGE

Calming and soothing to the nervous system, Front Lunge dispels fatigue and refreshes the brain. The leg muscles are toned and strengthened. This pose can be helpful in relieving depression and stress-related headaches and migraines. If you have low blood pressure, come out of the pose gradually to avoid dizziness. Front Lunge is best done on a yoga mat. Keep your eyes open to maintain your balance.

Poses that bring the head down below the heart are calming for the mind. Incorporating this pose into your practice can help to reduce fatigue, improve focus, and lift the stress and anxiety that contribute to depression.

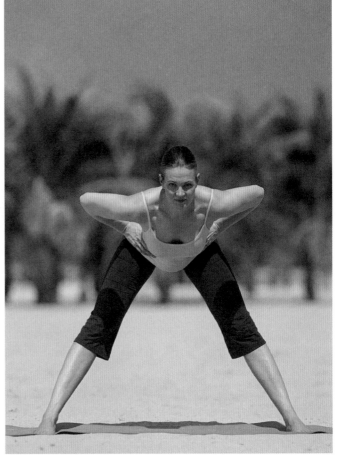

(1) Stand straight with your feet straddled about 4 ft (1.2 m) apart. Place your hands on your hips and inhale.

(2) As you start to exhale, bring your body forward until it is parallel to the ground. Keep your back straight, your head facing forward, and your chin up. Use your abdominal muscles to support your spine in this position.

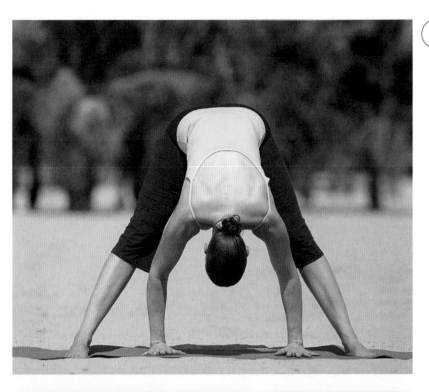

3 Place your hands on the ground in front of you, fingers spread and arms about shoulder-width apart. Press your hips upward and backward, moving your weight slightly toward your heels. Take a few breaths in this position.

4 Move your hands closer to your body, with the fingertips touching the ground. Lift your chin and lengthen your spine as you flatten your back, inhale, and then exhale. Continue on to step 5.

▶

⑤ Inhale and raise your arms evenly out to the sides, with your palms out straight; your fingers together, thumbs extended; and your back flat. Breathe deeply and hold for a few breaths.

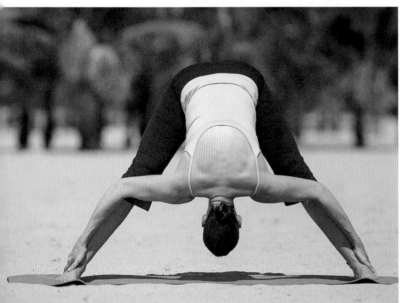

⑥ Relax your head and upper body downward while exhaling slowly, bringing your arms down and clasping your ankles or heels, whichever you can reach comfortably. Lengthen your spine and stretch your head toward the ground. Breathe normally and hold for a few breaths.

⑦ To come out of the pose, bring your hands to the ground in front of you, bend your elbows and knees slightly, and with a small jump, bring your legs back together as you inhale. Bend your knees in a squatting position, then stand up.

MEDITATION FOR EMOTIONAL BALANCE

Although this meditation is for everyone, it can be particularly good for a woman when she feels overly sensitive, worried, upset, or on the verge of anger.

Before practicing this meditation, drink a glass of filtered water, preferably at room temperature. Emotions and the need for water are intricately connected. When there is an imbalance of water in the system and the kidneys are pressurized, there is a tendency toward anxiety and upset behavior. From a scientific point of view, water is the medium that increases electrical potential across cell membranes, which is essential for the proper functioning of the nervous system.

The combination of drinking water, followed by applying pressure at the armpits with the raised shoulders and a Neck Lock, creates a tight lock on the entire upper body. Combined with a natural slowing of the breathing rate, this locked posture forms an automatic "brake" that is applied to the brain. The brain cannot continue its previous pattern of thinking, and within a short amount of time, a balance is restored. Those with high blood pressure, a neck injury, or heart disease should consult with their physician before practicing this meditation.

1 Sit in Easy pose. If necessary, place a firm pillow, bolster, or thick blanket under your buttocks to allow the knees to relax down so that you are comfortable. Straighten the spine and relax the shoulders. Keep the chest lifted throughout the meditation. Place your arms across your chest and lock your hands under your armpits with the palms open and against the body. The thumbs may be outside the armpits. Close your eyes.

2 Raise your shoulders up toward your ear lobes as far as possible and hold them there. Apply a Neck Lock by contracting back on the neck and throat. The chin is pulled back toward the neck without tipping the head forward. If you are doing it correctly, you will feel that the cervical vertebrae are in alignment with the spine. Stay alert throughout the meditation to maintain the Neck Lock and raised shoulders, which are the essential components of the "brake" you are applying to the brain. Your breath will automatically become slower.

Begin with 3 minutes of meditation, gradually increasing the time to 11 minutes.

BREAST CARE

Among the women who come to my yoga classes, there are typically one or two breast cancer survivors and often at least one woman who is in the midst of dealing with breast cancer. Keeping our breasts healthy is one of the most important things we can do. One of the best ways is to activate the lymphatic system, which—in addition to helping your body fight infection—removes potentially harmful materials from the body's tissues and cells. Lymph flow is dependent upon muscle contractions, which massage the outside of the lymphatic vessels, and breathing, which pulls lymph along with each inhalation. With its sensitivity to breathing and movement, it is easy to see how the lymph system responds very positively to yoga practice.

HEALTHY BREASTS

The following simple yoga exercises stimulate the circulation of blood and vital energy through the lymphatic system. Feel free to practice these exercises and postures individually or as a set. The first two, Diagonal Stretch and Reach for Health, can be done either sitting on the floor or on a chair with the spine straight and the feet flat on the floor.

The endocrine system, which includes hormones and glands, is balanced through yoga. This is important with regard to the breasts since estrogen must be in balance with its partner hormone, progesterone, in order to function properly.

DIAGONAL STRETCH

In this exercise, the lymphatic system is activated by vigorous movement and powerful breathing. The pad at the base of the little finger is a reflex point that empowers the communication center of the brain.

① Sit in Easy pose (p.19). Place your thumbs on the pads of the hands at the base of your little fingers. Keep the rest of the fingers straight. Extend your arms out to the sides, parallel to the ground, with the palms facing downward.

② Alternately raise one arm up 60° from the horizontal while bringing the other arm down 60°. Inhale as the left arm goes up, and exhale as the right arm goes up. Breathe powerfully and move quickly. Continue for 1–3 minutes.

REACH FOR HEALTH

In this exercise, the powerful movement of the arms, coupled with the forceful breath, is similar to a martial arts exercise. The "snapping back" movement activates the lymph and breast tissue.

Other yoga postures that benefit the lymph/breast area are Bow, Cobra, and Shoulderstand.

① Sit on your heels. If you need to take pressure off the knee joints, place a firm pillow between your buttocks and legs. Make your hands into fists with your thumbs tucked inside. Bring your hands to chest level with your arms by your sides, elbows pulled back.

② Powerfully extend one arm forward on a deep inhalation. As your arm extends to its full length, open your fingers as though you were grasping something. Then close them quickly, again with the thumb inside, and snap the arm back powerfully to the side of your body as you exhale strongly. Repeat with the other arm and continue this sequence for 1–2 minutes.

JUMP FOR HEALTH

Jumping on a rebounder, or mini trampoline, greatly improves the circulation of lymphatic fluid within the body, which in turn improves the body's cancer-fighting ability. To help your lymph system, jump and jog while moving your arms up and down and in circles. Lively, uplifting music will give you a rhythm to rebound to, and singing along will expand your lung capacity and just generally help you feel wonderfully alive. (See also Music Resources, p.224, for suggestions on suitable music.)

FROG POSE

This exercise increases the flow of energy to the body and mind. Internal heat (called tapas) and energy move from the pelvic area upward through the heart center and balance the glandular system.

Fold the body forward as much as possible

(1) While standing, bring your heels close together, or touching, and turn your feet slightly outward. Squat down, keeping your heels off the ground and bringing your fingertips to the ground with the arms inside your spread knees. Straighten your spine as much as possible in this squatting position.

(2) Inhale and straighten the legs, bringing the head as close to the knees as you can. The fingertips remain on the ground and the heels stay slightly off the ground. Exhale and return to squatting position. Continue for 1–3 minutes, then relax.

ONE-LEGGED BOW

This exercise stretches and increases circulation under the arms where the lymph system is active. One-Legged Bow pose also stimulates the glandular system.

1 Lie down on your front with your arms resting at your sides and your feet slightly apart.

2 Bend one leg toward your head and grasp the foot with hands interlaced, or one hand on top of the other. If you cannot reach the ankle, loop a belt around the ankle and grasp either end of the belt.

3 Create a tension between the arms and the leg and arch the body up in One-Legged Bow pose.

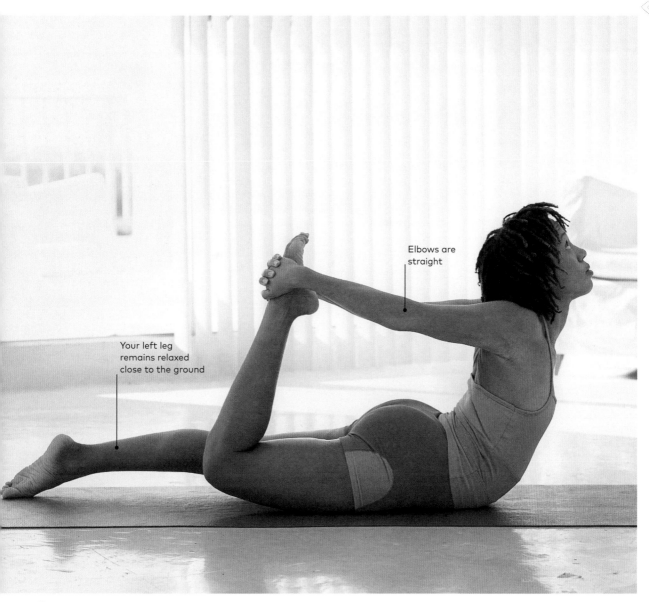

Elbows are
straight

Your left leg
remains relaxed
close to the ground

4 Inhale as you lift yourself higher and rock back
onto your pelvis, arching your upper spine,
expanding your chest, and lifting your head.

▶

(5) Exhale as you rock forward onto the upper chest, keeping the arms straight and the leg arched high. Your chin may come to the ground. The leg that is on the ground is straight and will move slightly off the ground with the rocking movement. Continue rocking back and forth with strong breaths for 1 minute, then switch legs and repeat for another minute.

(6) Rest for at least 20 seconds with the head turned to one side and your arms relaxed by your sides, palms facing up.

DRY BRUSH MASSAGE

One-third of the body's impurities are eliminated through the skin. Dry-brush massage stimulates the lymphatic system to expel toxins through the skin and allows the skin to breathe more efficiently. Using a long-handled natural bristle brush or loofah mitt, start with the soles of your feet and then move upward. Brush with as much pressure as is comfortable until your skin feels pleasantly warm. Continue for about 5 minutes. The face and ears can be brushed with a soft facial brush. Follow with a brief cold shower (p.33) or contrast shower (alternating warm and cold water) to increase the cleansing effects.

BEAUTIFUL BREASTS

Our breasts don't have to sag with the passage of time if we know what to do to keep the supporting muscles strong. Just think how much healthier your breasts can be when they are able to support themselves with their own muscles rather than relying on "supportive" but tight bras, which can seriously constrict your vital circulation. Here are a few exercises to keep your breasts firm and healthy.

In his book, *Breast Health: A Ten Point Prevention Program*, Dr. Charles Simone outlines a plan for breast care: optimize nutrition; take antioxidant supplements; and avoid tobacco, alcohol, and estrogens. Exercise, minimize stress, become spiritually involved, and increase your awareness of your sexuality. Have regular physical examinations from the age of 35.

PALM PRESS

This strengthens the muscles around the breasts and those of the chest and upper arms. Press with as much pressure as you can. When you maintain this lifted posture during the day, you will notice that it is also uplifting for your mind.

Sitting in Easy pose (p.19) or standing, simply bring the palms of your hands together at chest level and press them together tightly as you exhale. Relax the pressure as you inhale, then begin again. Repeat 20 times or more.

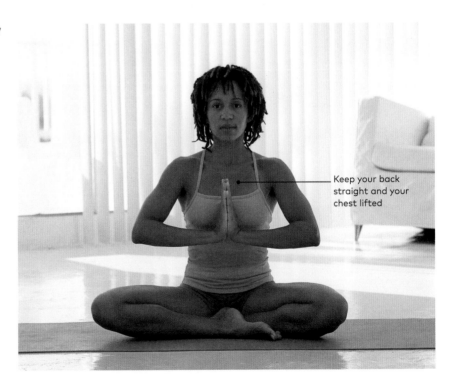

Keep your back straight and your chest lifted

ARM PRESS

This exercise strengthens the muscles around the breasts and the sides of the torso. It also strengthens the nervous system. Press with the maximum amount of pressure for the most benefit and repeat as often as you remember throughout the day.

Sitting in Easy pose or standing, place your palms and forearms together slightly above chest level. Lift your elbows a few inches away from your body. Press the entire length of the palms and forearms together on the exhalation. Inhale and release the press. Repeat 20 times or more.

WALL PRESS

This strengthens and tones the muscles of the chest and upper back. It is also beneficial for the abdominal and leg muscles, especially the calves and Achilles tendon in the heels. The inward-facing hand positions provide optimal benefit to the muscles around the breasts.

① Stand with your feet on the floor 24–28 in (45–60 cm) away from the wall. Place your hands on the wall about shoulder-width apart, with the arms positioned so that the elbows are facing outward and the fingers of each hand face inward toward each other. Inhale.

② As you exhale, bend your elbows and bring your nose toward the wall. On the inhalation, return to the original position. Bend only the elbows, keeping the legs straight. Continue for 10–20 repetitions.

LOVING & MOTHERING

Loving starts with yourself, as does mothering. You've got to have something before you have something to give. In this section, you'll find yoga to empower your womanly spirit, helping it to bend without breaking in the face of life's challenges.

Quite often, our biggest challenges are about how we relate to and care for those we love most—our partners and our children—which can often bring out painful emotions. The yoga here not only helps you gain perspective and balance with these strong emotional ties, but also helps to free up your ability to create the family life you want—and have fun in the meantime.

SELF-EMPOWERMENT

Ancient yogic wisdom speaks of the mythological figure Shakti, the divine feminine, as the creative power and principle of existence itself. Without Shakti, nothing can manifest or bloom. Woman is said to be made in the image of Shakti. She represents that very same creative energy on the earth. Simply put, woman equals power.

This chapter contains yoga and meditation to empower you in every way, including the ability to create a life of prosperity. True prosperity translates into every area of your life: physically, you are robust and healthy; spiritually, you enjoy life and share your abundance with others; and materially, you are successful and have the resources you need.

SET FOR SHAKTI ENERGY

This is a workout on every level: mind, body, and spirit. It is an aerobic set that strengthens three important systems: glandular, immune, and nervous systems. As you chant, the tongue strikes the upper palate, stimulating the hypothalamus—the master gland that controls the mind-body connection. This set empowers your sense of self and helps you feel light and blissful. Meditation afterward is effortless.

Each part of this set consists of eight movements coordinated with eight repetitions of the mantra *Har* (the Infinite). Roll the "r" off the roof of your mouth so that *Har* sounds like "hudah" (short "u," as in hut). Feel your belly naturally come inward each time you chant *Har*. This activates the third chakra, your point of personal power. The set has 11 continuous exercises, which are repeated. Start with 5–10 rounds and work up to as many as possible without overexerting yourself.

1 OVERHEAD CLAP

This pose stretches the spine and stimulates the meridian points in the hands, which activate brain clarity. The lymphatic areas of the arms and chest are stimulated, promoting good breast health.

(1) Stand straight with the feet shoulder-width apart, weight evenly distributed on all parts of the feet. Extend your arms straight up overhead so that the arms are close to your ears.

(2) Firmly clap the entire surface of the palms together eight times, chanting *Har* each time.

2 STRIKE THE GROUND

Forward bending relaxes and stretches the spine and invigorates the mind and nervous system. Clapping the ground stimulates meridian points in the hands that connect to the brain and improve your mental clarity.

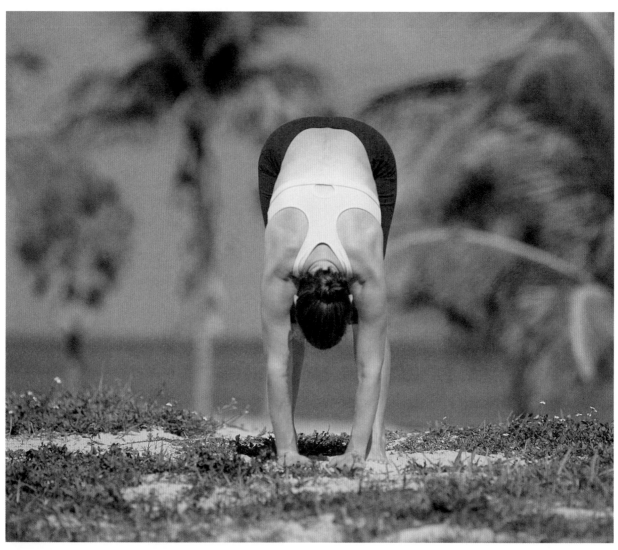

Following the Overhead Clap, immediately bend forward, keeping the arms close to the ears. Strike the ground with your palms eight times, chanting *Har*. Make sure that your knees are not locked. If you cannot reach the ground, bend your knees slightly.

3 ARM FLAPS

In this exercise, the lymphatic areas are stimulated, promoting good breast health. Keeping the arms straight activates reflex points associated with the colon, stomach, spleen, and liver, and tension is released from the shoulders.

① After Strike the Ground, straighten the spine and come back into a standing position. Bring your arms out to the sides of your body at shoulder level, parallel to the ground. Your fingers are straight with the palms facing downward.

② Begin flapping your arms without bending the elbows. Move approximately 6 in (15 cm) up and down from the horizontal in one smooth motion. Each time your arms move up or down, chant *Har* for a total of eight times.

4 CRISS-CROSS

This is the aerobic section of this yoga set, which strengthens the heart, glands, and metabolism. If you need to go at a more gentle pace, step the feet into and out of the criss-cross position instead of jumping. Alternate the crossing of arms and legs.

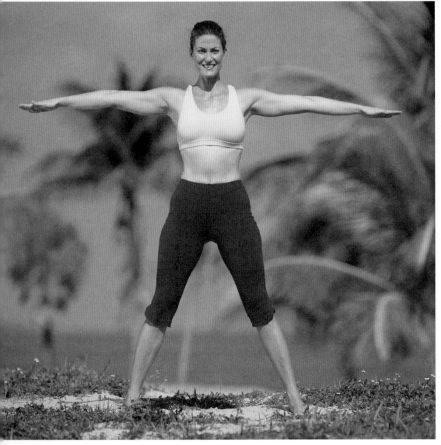

① Keep your arms extended out to the sides with the palms facing downward, parallel to the ground. Your feet should be slightly wider than shoulder-width apart.

The arms remain as straight as possible

② Bend your knees slightly as you jump and cross your legs. At the same time, cross your arms in front of your heart center. Chant *Har* as you cross and uncross the legs and arms eight times.

5 ARCHER

This pose helps to maintain the mineral balance of the body, especially that of calcium, magnesium, sodium, and potassium. It strengthens the electromagnetic energy field and improves concentration. Archer pose activates and balances all of your chakras and helps you develop courage.

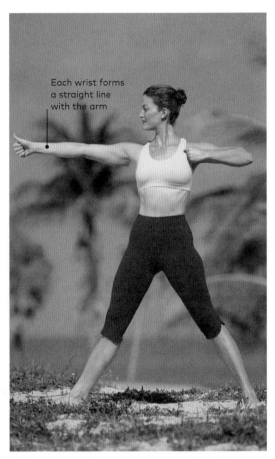

Each wrist forms a straight line with the arm

① Stand with your legs straddled about 30 in (75 cm) apart, with your right leg forward and your left leg back at a 45° angle to the front foot. Extend your arms out parallel to the ground.

② Raise your right arm straight in front of you. Make your right hand into a fist, as if grasping a bow, while pressing your thumb forward. Bring your left arm back as if pulling a bow string back to the shoulder, expanding and lifting the chest. Your left forearm is parallel to the ground, your hand in a fist, again with the thumb pressed forward.

▶

③ Bend the right knee so that the heel and knee are in line. Keep the body centered with the back leg stable and the front leg bearing more of the weight. Face forward and fix your eyes past your outstretched arm, gazing at the horizon. Begin to pulse forward into the front leg and release slightly eight times, chanting *Har* each time.

④ Without breaking the rhythm of the exercise, pivot around on your feet so that your left leg and arm are forward and the right leg is back. Repeat the pulsing movement while chanting *Har* eight times. Repeat the criss-cross jumps (p.148) eight times while chanting *Har*.

6 BACKWARD STRETCH

This stretch invigorates and flexes the entire spine, including the cervical vertebrae. Stretching the arms activates the lymphatic system, promoting good breast health.

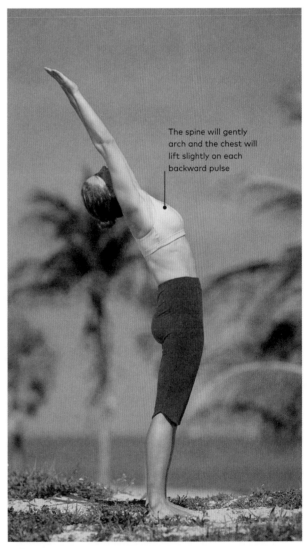

The spine will gently arch and the chest will lift slightly on each backward pulse

① With the feet shoulder-width apart, stretch the arms up overhead, arching the spine slightly back. Look upward toward your hands the entire time.

② Chant *Har* as you pulse the arms back, then release slightly, continuing eight times. The spine will gently arch and the chest lift slightly on each pulse. Repeat the criss-cross jumps (p.148) eight times while chanting *Har*.

7 SIDE STRETCHES

These lateral stretches improve spinal flexibility, stimulate the lymphatic system, increase muscle tone, and aid digestion. This is the only exercise with a count of four on each side, totaling eight repetitions.

This is the last yoga pose of the set. Begin the set again on p.145 and repeat the entire series 5–25 times.

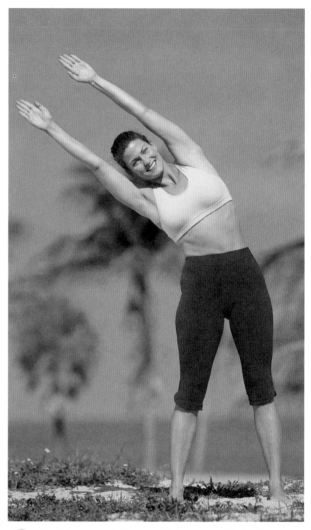

① Stretch the arms up overhead. Bend directly to the right side so that a lateral stretch is created on the left side of the body. Make sure not to bend forward or back, but directly to the side.

② Begin to pulse and release slightly for a count of 4, chanting *Har* each time. Without stopping, stretch to the left side for four counts. Repeat the criss-cross jumps (p.148) eight times while chanting *Har*.

8 TO END

After doing this set for an extended period of time, it is important to rest. If you practice it on consecutive days, alternate between the following positions for relaxation: on one day, rest on your back with the knees pulled into the chest and the arms wrapped around the bent legs. The next day, rest in Child's pose (p.50). Relax for at least 5 minutes—preferably more—and listen to an uplifting piece of music (see also p.224).

ADI SHAKTI MEDITATION

This meditation uses the Kundalini Bhakti mantra, the "female power." It describes four qualities of the feminine aspect of creative power: the power that gave birth to all creation, the power that is forever, the power that cuts through darkness, and the nurturing power of the mother. It can be chanted powerfully from the heart center in a monotone, or sung (see also Music Resources, p.224).

The mantra has four parts:

1 *Adi Shakti, Adi Shakti, Adi Shakti, Namo Namo* (Ah-dee Shah-k tee, Nah-moe) meaning, "To the primal power that creates all things, I bow."

2 *Sarab Shakti, Sarab Shakti, Sarab Shakti, Namo Namo* (Sah-rub Shah-k tee) meaning, "To the total power of Shakti, I bow."

3 *Prithum Bagwati, Prithum Bagwati, Prithum Bagwati, Namo Namo* (Prit-um Bah-g wut-ee) meaning, "To the original Goddess, The Sword of Truth, I bow."

4 *Kundalini, Mata Shakti, Mata Shakti, Namo Namo* (Kun-da-leen-ee, Mah-tah Shah-k tee) meaning, "To the Kundalini, the mother power, I bow."

Sit in Easy pose, spine straight, chest lifted, and chin slightly tucked back toward the neck. Suggested mudras are: hands in the lap; right palm resting inside the left; tips of the thumbs touching; or arms crossed over the heart center with the left palm underneath and right over the left. Close your eyes and vibrate the mantra from your heart. Feel the navel pull in slightly with the rhythm. Feel the energy of Shakti within you and all around you as you chant for 5, 11, or 31 minutes.

RELEASING FEAR & ANGER

I gratefully count myself among the many women
who have found yoga and meditation to work
wonders when it comes to strong emotions such
as fear and anger. I think of yoga and meditation
as partners, my two best friends, who upon
finding me in a drama or trauma roll up their
sleeves and get right into the mess with me. They
are loyal friends who help me get out all my
"stuff," see it for what it is, then efficiently and
effectively help me clean it up and send it on its
way. My load lightened, I am left with tons of
gratitude and a renewed dedication to my yoga
practice. The yoga and meditation exercises
in this chapter, and in this entire book, serve
as a means toward that end.

KUNDALINI SALUTATIONS

This set of postures and exercises strengthens and tones the muscles, releases fear and anger, and elevates the consciousness. It is called Kundalini Salutations because it works to awaken the kundalini energy. Once awakened, this energy provides you with the awareness you need to live to your full potential.

1 UPPER TORSO LIFTS

This pose opens up the meridians of the abdomen, solar plexus, heart center, and throat, which are associated with the navel chakra (seat of power and passion), heart chakra (home of altruistic love and compassion), and the throat chakra (ability to speak truth).

The yogic numbers 26, 54, and 108 are cycles that have particular effects on your body and mind. Begin with 26 or 54 repetitions and, with practice, move on to 108.

① Lie on your abdomen with your chin on the ground and interlace your hands behind your back. For wrist problems, try grasping your wrists or a short rope or belt instead.

② As you inhale, raise your upper torso off the ground as high as possible, using your abdominal, upper chest, and back muscles. Stretch your arms back and up simultaneously, as high as you can without straining. Exhale and relax the body back down with a rolling motion, keeping your hands clasped behind your back.

Count out loud to maintain your focus

2 ROCKING BOW

This helps regulate a woman's hormones, which play a primary role in her emotional balance. If rocking is difficult, try lifting the body on the inhalation (as in step 4) and relaxing down on the exhalation (as in step 5).

Dynamic asanas such as Rocking Bow tone and revitalize the internal organs and bring balance to the body's hormones.

1. Lie on your abdomen with your arms at your sides, palms facing upward and chin on the ground.

2. Raise your head up off the ground. Bend your right leg at the knee and reach back with your right hand to grasp the ankle.

3. Bend your left leg at the knee and grab the ankle with your left hand. Keep the legs as close together as possible. If you cannot reach your ankles, loop a belt around your feet and hold onto the two sides of the belt as close to your feet as possible (see also p.47).

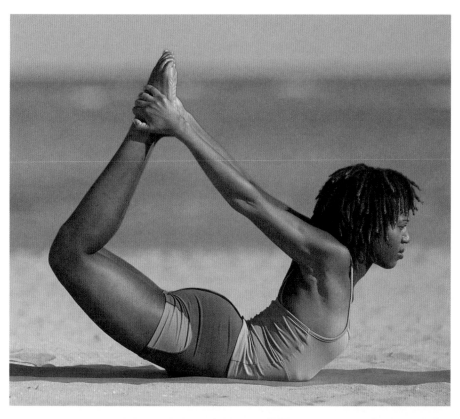

④ Inhale and lift your body upward, raising your head, chest, and thighs up off the ground. Create a tension between the straight arms and the legs to stretch up higher without straining. Your elbows remain straight. Use your upper body strength to stretch up. Look straight ahead. Prepare yourself to exhale and rock forward.

⑤ As you exhale, rock forward so that your head comes down and your thighs lift off the ground as much as possible without you straining.

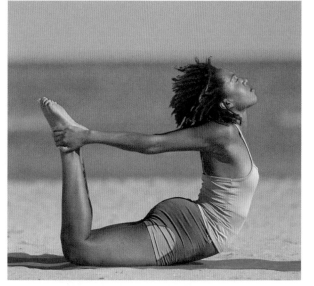

⑥ Inhale as you rock back and your chest lifts up. Continue Rocking Bow, counting up to 26, 54, or 108 as you rock. Each forward and backward movement counts as one.

3 BOWING POSE

This pose generates internal heat, or tapas, from the base of the spine to the base of the neck. As you bow with arms outstretched, the lymph area under the armpits is stimulated. Be aware of touching your third eye point (located between the eyebrows) to the ground as you bow; this creates a natural focal point for the mind.

① Sit on your heels with a straight spine. Press the palms of your hands together in Prayer pose (p.22), then bring them to the center of your chest so that the thumbs press against the breastbone. Inhale deeply in this position.

② As you exhale, bend forward, and in one smooth motion bring your torso and your hands down to the ground. As you bow with your hands in Prayer pose, slide the outside edges of your hands forward until your arms are stretched out straight and your forehead touches the ground. Perform this pose 26, 54, or 108 times.

4 JUMP AROUND

Jumping your body in this way strengthens your nervous system and releases tension and anxiety. Make sure you have a soft surface underneath you before practicing this exercise. Then have fun with it!

Lie down on your back with your arms at your sides, palms facing downward. Begin to freely jump your body all around. Press your legs and arms against the ground to jump your torso. Move your legs and arms. Move your head and neck from side to side, taking care not to jerk or bump your head against the ground. Continue for 1–3 minutes.

5 SITALI COBRA

Sitali breath, the Sanskrit name for Cooling breath (p.77), cools off anger, soothes the nervous system, and calms anxiety and fear. Coupled with the Cobra pose, it stimulates the pranic flow of energy throughout the spine and torso, distributing vital energy to the entire body and mind.

1 Lie down on your abdomen with your body relaxed. Place your hands on the ground on either side of your chest, keeping the elbows in close to your sides.

2 As you begin to lift into Cobra pose, inhale using the Sitali breath: extend your tongue and curl the sides upward (inset). Draw cool air in through your rolled tongue as you inhale.

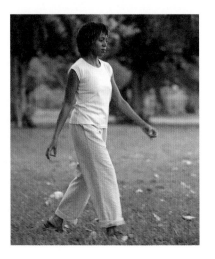

WALKING MEDITATION

A fun and effective form of meditation can be done by walking in rhythm as you breathe, inhaling to the count of two or four steps and exhaling for the same length of time. Or add a mantra: try chanting Sa Ta Na Ma while pressing your fingers (p.97). You may chant silently or out loud. Keep your gaze in front of you to maintain your meditative state. The yogic science of walking meditation is called Breathwalk and has helped many people reduce stress and increase calmness just by the simple act of walking (see Resources).

Inhale through
your rolled tongue
and exhale through
the nose

③ At the same time, stretch back into Cobra using your upper chest and
abdominal muscles, as well as your arms, to lift up and curve back.

④ Close your mouth and exhale through your
nose as you return to the ground. Pay
special attention to uncurling your spine
so that your abdomen rests on the ground
first, followed by your upper chest, neck,
and then head. Continue to inhale up into
Cobra using the Sitali breath, then exhale
down, breathing out through the nose.

⑤ After 1½ minutes, relax with your head
turned to one side, or come into Child's
pose (p.50) by sitting back on your heels
with your forehead on the ground and
your arms relaxed by your sides.

6 MANTRA MEDITATION

In this meditation at the end of the set, you learn to direct an internal sound into your chakras using your imagination. The result is that you become more self-aware and in control of your thoughts and actions. Start off with one repetition of the mantra on the held inhalation and exhalation. As you become familiar with this process, try to repeat the mantra three times or more on each inhalation and exhalation.

After this, sing along to the music "Naad: The Blessing" (see music resources, p.224) or sit silently for 3 minutes, then relax on your back for 10 minutes.

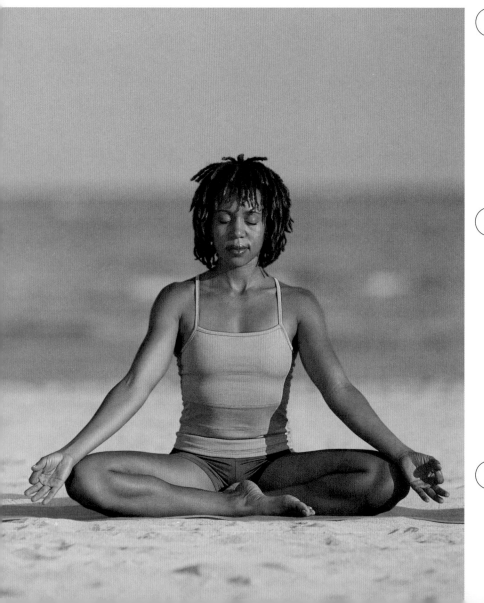

① Sit in Easy pose. Straighten the lower vertebrae, lift the chest, and draw the chin slightly in toward the neck to bring the cervical vertebrae in line with the spine. Rest your hands on your knees in passive Gyan Mudra (p.21), first finger and thumb touching and the other fingers extended but relaxed. Close your eyes.

② Inhale deeply and hold your breath. Mentally chant the mantra *Har Har Wahe Guru:* pull your navel slightly toward your spine and upward as you mentally sound *Har* (rhymes with "car") at your navel point, then sound *Har* at your heart center. Mentally project the sound *Wa* ("la") at your throat center, then *He* ("hey") at your brow point, or intuitive center. Finally, imagine the sound *Guru* ("gu-roo") at the top of your head.

③ Repeat the mantra mentally as many times as you can on the held inhalation, then exhale and hold the breath out, repeating the same process. Continue for 11 minutes.

PRANAYAMA TO EXPEL NEGATIVITY AND DISEASE

This pranayama, or breathing exercise, uses the circle breath, which cleanses out whatever is the root of the problem within you. It has a purgative effect, ridding your body of disease and your mind of anger, sorrow, and fear. On the four-part inhalation, your lungs will fill in one continuous motion as follows:

On the initial part of the inhalation, the lowest part of the lungs are filled and the abdomen expands outward.

On the second part, the lower rib cage expands.

On the third, the chest begins to expand.

On the last part of the inhalation, the top of the chest is filled with the breath and the throat and shoulders feel an expansion.

1 Sit up straight in Easy pose. Bend your right arm up at the elbow and bring it close to the side of your body with your open palm facing forward, as though you are taking an oath. Then raise your left arm with the elbow bent and bring the forearm around in front of the chest, parallel to the ground, with the fingers straight and the palm facing down. Keep your eyes closed. Form an "o" shape with your mouth and begin to inhale powerfully and deeply in four distinct parts (see above). Then exhale with one long breath. Continue for 11–22 minutes.

2 To end the pranayama, inhale as deeply as you can, relaxing your diaphragm and opening up the chest cavity. Hold your breath and stretch your arms up straight and as high possible, with your fingers spread wide and as tight as steel. Stretch your entire spine upward. Exhale strongly through the mouth like firing a cannon. Repeat two more times, then relax.

Step 1   Step 2

"People who do breathing exercises will have the capacity for very long breaths. They will have extra prana …. If prana is less in you, then you are less in you."
Yogi Bhajan

RELATIONSHIPS

Every challenge, every conflict, every dream, and every prayer that you have comes from you and is resolved by you. It all comes back to you. Nowhere is this more apparent than in relationships with your partner. Other chapters in this book help you to be a woman who is solidly prepared for enlightened relationships. This chapter will help you blend your male and female sides and strengthen your inner resolve. Partner yoga and meditations allow your energies to blend and your hearts to open up to each other. This chapter is also the place to turn to when you are not getting along in your relationships or when there is discord, dissatisfaction, or disappointment.

VENUS KRIYAS

Venus (meaning love) Kriyas are exercises that are shared between partners. The internal energy is drawn and directed positively toward subconscious cleansing and the raising of energy through the chakras to higher consciousness. Each of the kriyas is complete in itself; choose just one or two to do and practice each for no longer than 3 minutes. Begin by tuning in (p.22).

GETTING RID OF GRUDGES

When you and your partner have felt discord between you, whether spoken or not, this exercise helps you both to clear the air between you and start over fresh. All it takes is a willingness to practice.

If your partner is willing to join you, be grateful. If not, be grateful anyway. You'll feel happy, and happiness is contagious. Your partner may be curious about what's making you feel so good.

Sit back to back with your partner, with the length of your spines touching. Put your feet flat on the floor in front of you, bring your knees up, and wrap your arms around them. Close your eyes and breathe. Meditate on your heart—hear it and feel it. Meditate on the sun, bringing it into your heart. Burn out all the bitterness and grudges that you may have been carrying. Continue for 3 minutes.

SENDING PRANA

In this exercise, you use your hands and eyes to energize each other and build a healing energy between you. Keeping the arms straight increases nerve strength in the arms and pranic energy in the hands.

Each partner's palms should be flat with the fingers straight

The arms and spine are also straight

Sit on your heels in Rock pose (p.20). Stretch your arms out at shoulder level so that your palms touch those of your partner. Gaze into each other's eyes, blinking as little as possible. Feel that you are sending prana to each other through your hands and eyes. Experience this sensation. Continue for 2 minutes, then close your eyes and visualize your partner for 1 minute more.

CROW SQUATS

Crow Squats benefit your hips, lower spine, and leg muscles by opening, stretching, and toning them. Energy in the lower chakras is stimulated and circulated to the upper chakras. This exercise can be aerobic and heart-strengthening.

1 Stand facing your partner with your feet shoulder-width apart. You may have to adjust your feet in order to maintain balance while squatting. Join hands and look into each other's eyes with love. Verbally greet each other, then continue talking to each other throughout the exercise.

2 Bend your knees and squat down together so that your buttocks are close to the ground. Ideally your feet will be flat on the ground. Your body will naturally lean forward a bit, but keep the spine as straight as possible. Return to standing and continue for 3 minutes. If possible, each complete up-and-down cycle should take 4 seconds. Those with medical conditions should exert caution and move slowly. Half-knee bends may be done by those with knee problems.

HEART LOTUS

This kriya slows you down from your busy daily lives and brings an awareness of the shared heart. Adjust your height using a pillow if you cannot comfortably see into each other's eyes.

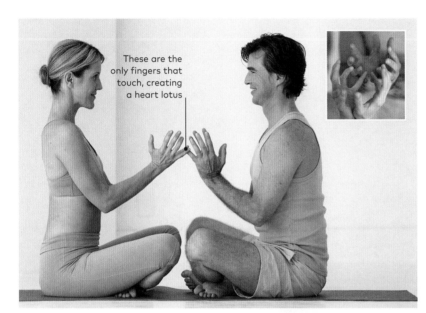

These are the only fingers that touch, creating a heart lotus

1. Sit in Easy pose (p.19) with your knees almost touching. Put the base of your hands and wrists together and spread the hands to form a lotus flower (inset). The man positions his little fingers under those of the woman. Look into the soul of your partner through their eyes for 1–1½ minutes.

2. Place one hand over the other at your heart center. Close your eyes and meditate on your heart. Go deep within to the center of your being. Continue the meditation for 1–1½ minutes. Then inhale and exhale deeply three times, relax the posture, and thank your partner.

COUPLES' KUNDALINI LOTUS

This exercise helps channel sexual energy and maintain potency and brings depth and lightness to your relationship. It requires flexibility, so warm up with Spine Flex (pp.31–32) and Spread Stretch (pp.36–37) first.

① Sit fairly close across from each other and hold hands. With the legs positioned outside the arms, bend the knees and place the bottoms of your feet and your partner's feet together. Lean back slightly, straightening the arms.

② Slowly stretch the legs up straight to a 60° angle from the ground, with the soles of the feet touching. Look into each other's eyes with love and joy. See yourself in the other person. Lift your partner's energy with your love, and realize that you two are one.

Continue for 3 minutes with either Breath of Fire or long, deep breathing. (Decide before you start which type of breathing you wish to do; both partners should do the same.) Then relax.

FOR INTERNAL STRENGTH

These individual exercises and poses have been chosen for their ability to build balance, endurance, and auric strength, which is essential for a woman whether she is single or in a relationship.

WARRIOR

A regular practice of Warrior pose develops an intensity of focus, mental strength, and endurance. It relieves cramps in the calves and thighs, brings elasticity to the leg and back muscles and makes the legs strong, and tones the abdominal organs. To prevent your bent knee from overworking and distribute the weight evenly, keep the knee directly over the ankle.

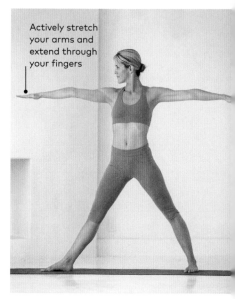

Actively stretch your arms and extend through your fingers

(1) Stand straight with your feet together. Bring your hands together in Prayer pose at the center of your chest and inhale.

(2) Exhale as you spread your legs 4 ft (1.2 m) apart, with your feet parallel and facing forward. Raise your arms to the sides in line with your shoulders, palms facing down and shoulders relaxed.

(3) Inhale and turn your right foot 90° to the right and your left foot slightly to the right. Keep your hips and chest facing forward while turning your head to the right. Slightly tighten the muscles around your left knee.

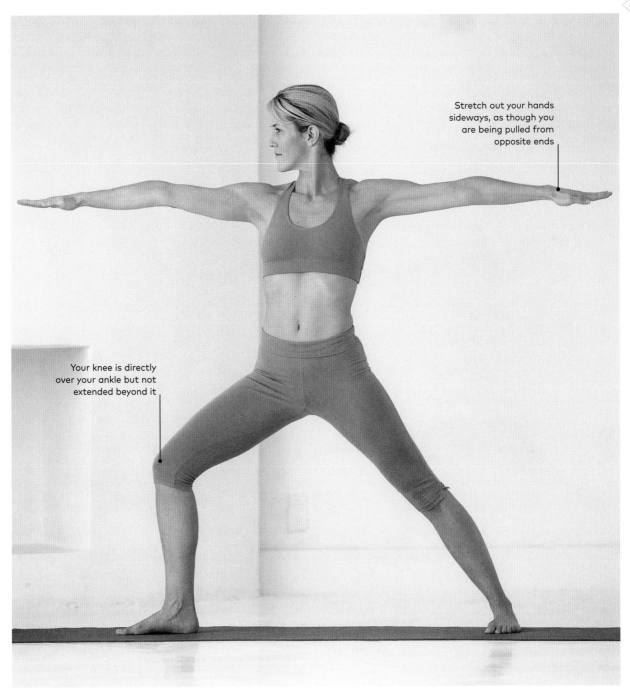

Stretch out your hands sideways, as though you are being pulled from opposite ends

Your knee is directly over your ankle but not extended beyond it

4　Exhale and bend your right knee until the thigh is nearly parallel to the ground and your knee is over your ankle. Turn your head and face to your right palm. Stretch the back muscles of your left leg fully. Breathe deeply for 1–2 minutes.

VARUYAS KRIYA

This kriya can cause a cleansing sweat. The amount of time spent practicing Varuyas Kriya can be slowly increased up to 7½ minutes on each side. There is a strong tendency to shake while practicing this pose as it adjusts and strengthens your nervous system. The practice and perfection of this kriya is said to improve the functioning of the pituitary gland, regulate excessive sexual energy, and increase general immunity to disease.

Similar in action and effect to Sat Kriya (pp.56–57), Varuyas (VAR-uh-yas) Kriya is a powerful, somewhat strenuous pose. You may want to stand on a yoga mat beside a wall for support in case you feel unsteady.

① Stand straight with your arms at your sides. Place the right leg as far back as you can while maintaining your balance. Bend your front leg so that your knee is bent directly over the foot but not extended beyond that point.

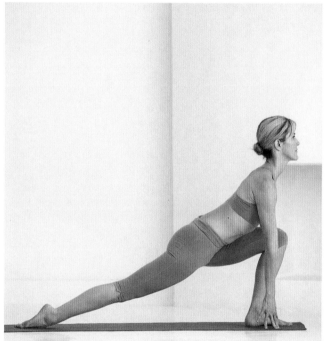

② Bring your hands to the ground by your front foot for balance. Place the top of your right foot on the ground so that the leg and foot extend out behind you in a straight line. Take a deep breath in.

The arms and hands form a straight line with the palms together, fingers pointing straight ahead, and thumbs side by side

Pull the navel point in and pull up slightly on the perineum

③ Exhale and extend the arms forward. The spine is extended slightly forward. Fix your eyes on the horizon and feel centered at the brow point. Begin chanting Sat Nam. Emphasize Sat (Truth) and apply a light Root Lock (p.25). On Nam (Identity), relax the muscular pull. Continue for 1–2 minutes. Then inhale, exhale, and relax, bending forward for a few seconds. Repeat with the right leg forward.

PREPARING
FOR BIRTH

Pregnancy is a most extraordinary time of
a woman's life: dramatic hormonal and bodily
changes week by week and even day by day can
make her life pretty topsy-turvy. Yoga provides
a calm sanctuary where she can experience a
peaceful, loving union with her baby; discover her
inner grit; and delve into the practice of breath
awareness. Yoga's primary gifts of increasing
flexibility and decreasing tension are perfectly
compatible with the needs of a pregnant woman.
Here are postures that open and relax the pelvic
area, strengthen muscle tone, and release back
tension, coupled with deep breathing and a
meditative focus to deepen your experience
of the life growing within you.

ACTIVE STANDING POSE

When you are pregnant, most of the extra weight you carry is all in one place. Because your abdominal muscles (which normally hold your lower torso in place) are missing in action, so to speak, you may develop a swayed back or exaggerated spinal curve. This can cause lower back pain and sciatica. Practice this pose as often as possible to lengthen your spine downward.

Be aware of any personal limitations in practicing pregnancy yoga. Consult your physician if necessary and stop exercises that cause discomfort. After the first trimester, avoid retaining the inhalation, abdominal exercises, those done lying on your front, and inverted poses (such as Downward Facing Dog, Plow, and Shoulderstand), and knee-to-chest positions. "Light" Breath of Fire may be practiced, but check with a physician first.

Relax and drop your shoulders, though maintain a slight lift to the chest. Stroke your lower back downward with your hands. Slightly drop your chin downward to relax the back of your neck. Breathe slowly for a minute.

PRENATAL POSES

The following poses are helpful during pregnancy. For example, poses done while kneeling on all fours will help to relieve back pain and strengthen back muscles, which aids labor. Because your pelvic floor supports the weight of your baby during pregnancy, squeezing the pelvic floor muscles (rectal and vaginal) to strengthen them should be done as often as possible, both on and off the mat.

CAT POSE

This exercise brings great flexibility to the spine (including the cervical vertebrae), circulates the spinal fluid, and serves as a great warm-up exercise. For added benefit, at the end of the exhalation, gently squeeze your buttock muscles for 1–2 seconds and then release as you inhale.

① Begin on your hands and knees with your knees directly under your hips and your hands under your shoulders. The hands, feet, and knees are in line with each other. Relax your neck and inhale, keeping your spine in a horizontal position. Do not arch your spine since this can put pressure on the lower back during pregnancy.

② As you exhale, lengthen the base of your spine gently downward and tuck your pelvis under so that your back is rounded like that of a cat. Inhale and return to the original position. If you experience pain in the wrists in this position, use your knuckles to support you so that your wrists remain straight.

BALANCING CAT

This posture is challenging and requires concentration. It develops balance and focus, both important areas for pregnancy and childbirth. For a good diagonal stretch, practice slowly with deep breaths.

(1) Begin on your hands and knees with your back horizontal. Keep your eyes open in a soft gaze to help maintain your balance.

(2) Inhale and raise your left arm out straight in front of you. At the same time, raise your right leg straight out behind you. Lift only as high as you can without arching your spine. Exhale and return your hand and leg to the ground. Inhale and raise the opposite arm and leg. Exhale and return to the original position. Continue for 1–2 minutes.

SUPPORTED BUTTERFLY

This pose helps to open the pelvis and hips and release tension from the area. This natural widening of the pelvis will help make it easier for your baby's head to engage in late pregnancy. Leaning back allows your lower back to relax and encourages the sacral vertebrae to self-adjust.

Hip-opening poses such as Supported Butterfly are beneficial in pregnancy, releasing tension in the pelvis to ensure comfort and opening up this area in preparation for the birth.

(1) Sit on the floor with the soles of your feet together. If you wish, use props for a more restful support (below).

Using props

Position your back support—either a beanbag or stack of bolsters, cushions, or thick blankets—at an angle similar to a chaise lounge and place a cushion under each knee.

(2) Put your hands behind you on the floor, or be supported by your props. Lean back, relaxing and stretching the spine. Relax your neck and shoulders, then your pelvis, hips, thighs, and knees. Breathe deeply for 1–2 minutes.

SQUATTING WITH A PARTNER

Squatting in childbirth is instinctive for a woman because it naturally allows the pelvis to open and the baby's head to engage. In the last 6 weeks of pregnancy, it is better to squat on a bolster to reduce pressure on the cervix and pelvic floor. Avoid squats if you have hemorrhoids, and check with your doctor first if you have a high-risk pregnancy.

Use a rolled towel under your heels if they do not reach the floor or a bolster for your bottom to rest on as you squat.

Squat down with or without the use of props. Make sure you are far enough away from your partner that both of you can have your arms out straight. Relax and breathe together with your partner for 1–2 minutes, then slowly stand up (inset) or come onto your hands and knees before standing up.

SQUAT WITH PRAYER POSE

This pose helps to increase your hip and pelvic flexibility by applying a moderate pressure against the knees. As you squat down, feel a gentle expansion in the hips. Check the cautions for squats on p.179.

Using props
Use several cushions for your bottom to rest on as you squat.

① Using props if needed (inset), squat down so that your buttocks are close to the ground. Bring your palms together in Prayer pose and rest the thumbs at the heart center in the middle of your chest. Your elbows will be out to the sides and touching the inside area of your knees. Inhale, then exhale and, with the elbows, exert a moderate pressure against the knees. Do this 5–10 times.

② Inhale deeply and exhale. Place your hands on the floor, straighten your legs, and slowly stand up. Alternatively, you can come onto your hands and knees as in step 1 of Cat pose (p.176) before standing up.

FORWARD BENDS

Practice these Forward Bends daily to release tension in the back,
stretch the muscles and nerves of the legs and arms, and relax
your shoulders. Do not practice if you feel dizzy or light-headed.

① Stand up straight with your legs about
shoulder-width apart, arms stretched
out in front, and facing a wall or table.

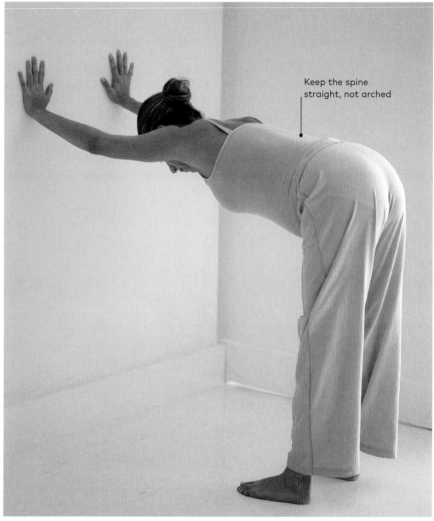

Keep the spine
straight, not arched

② Slowly exhale, lean forward, and put your hands on the wall—or hands and forearms on the table.
Allow the weight of your lower back to sink downward through your heels and into the floor.
Lengthen your spine without arching toward the floor. Let your neck relax. Feel a strong stretch
in the arms and legs. Breathe deeply for 1–2 minutes. Let your head relax forward and feel a
strong stretch in the arms and armpits. Breathe deeply for another 1–2 minutes.

EAR TO KNEE POSE

Besides being a great lateral stretch, this pose opens up much-needed breathing room in the lungs. Make sure you are stretching directly to either side of the body—you should avoid forward stretching after the first trimester since it puts pressure on the abdomen and womb.

① Sit with the legs extended and spine straight. Place your hands on the floor with fingers slightly spread. Then bend your right knee and tuck it in so that the foot is close to or against the inner thigh of the left leg.

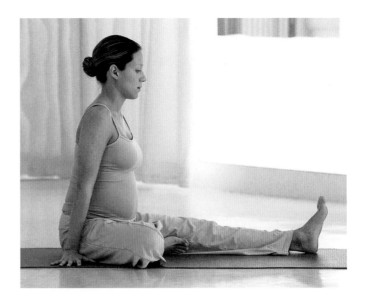

② Stretch your arms overhead. Exhale, keep your body facing forward, and stretch to the left, bringing your left ear toward your left knee as far as is comfortable. Rest your left arm on the ground inside your left leg. Breathe deeply and stretch for 3–5 breaths. Repeat on the right side. Continue for 1–2 minutes.

RESTING POSES

Relax in Side Lying or Front Lying pose as many times a day as possible, especially during the last few weeks of pregnancy, when you are fatigued from carrying extra weight or your sleep is often disturbed. Lying on your left side during the last 6 weeks will help to encourage your baby's spine toward the left side of your abdomen, which is the best position for labor. You may wish to vary this sometimes by lying on the right. Many women find the Side Lying position helpful for labor.

You will need several cushions, pillows, or folded blankets for these resting poses. Create enough height with the pillows so that the shoulder you lie on is not being crushed.

Side Lying
Lie on your left side on a soft surface with your head resting on a pillow. Extend your left leg out and then bend your right leg, placing a pillow or two under your right knee. Relax and breathe comfortably.

Front Lying
Lie on your left side on a soft surface with pillows placed under your head and bent knee. Face your upper body down toward the ground, extend your left arm downward by your side, and place your right arm upward by your head. Let your shoulders spread out and relax.

A THREE-WAY CONNECTION

Practice this exercise with your partner for a cozy feeling of togetherness. Share the space of love with your unborn child through voice, touch, massage, and meditation for as long as you both wish.

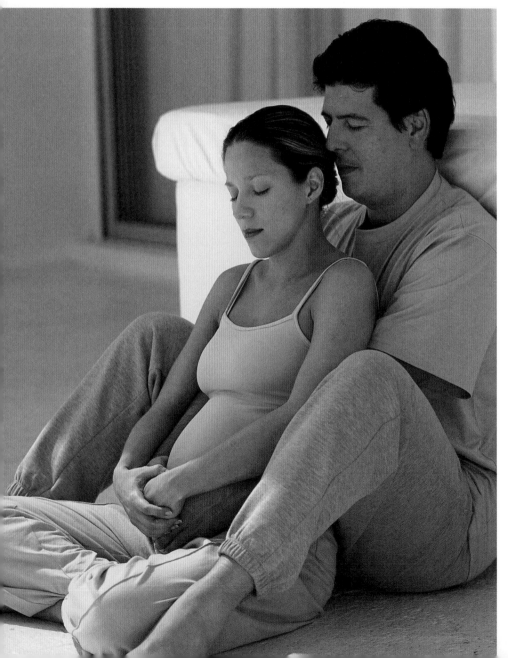

Have your partner sit against a wall with his legs apart and slightly out to the sides. Use pillows for support if desired. Let yourself get comfortable with your back resting against your partner's chest. Your partner's hands may rest on your abdomen with your hands on top. Cross your legs or leave them outstretched—whatever is comfortable. Focus on breathing together in a deep and relaxed manner. Let go of tension or tightness. Focus on the presence of your baby. Suggestions for a three-way connection are: stroking, feeling the energy of your hands surround and bless your child, or talking out loud or internally to your child.

SKIN CARE DURING PREGNANCY

Massage yogurt, lemon, and honey on the breasts, abdomen, and thighs once a week to prevent stretch marks, or take a yogurt bath (p.65). Oil your body regularly with a quality oil such as almond or sesame oil. Do not use soap on the nipples, as it dries the skin. If skin becomes dry or cracked, use the homeopathic salve Calendula. In preparation for breastfeeding, "toughen" up the nipples by squeezing and pinching them regularly, and rub well with a towel after bathing.

COMMUNING WITH YOUR UNBORN BABY

Make a special time in your day to sit with your baby, sending love and feeling the love your baby has for you. Your intuition, which is extra-strong during pregnancy, will lead you naturally to your favorite ways of communion with your baby. Perhaps this special connection happens during a sitting meditation early in the morning, as you sit in the rocking chair that you bought especially for nursing your baby, or as you float in a swimming pool while imagining your baby floating inside of you—whatever speaks to you as the most true way for you and your baby to connect.

Sit in Easy pose (p.19). Place your hands gently on your lower belly and cradle your baby. Close your eyes and let your head relax forward naturally. Focus on the rhythm of your breath and imagine how your baby experiences your heartbeat, your breath, and the sensation of floating in the warm fluid of your womb. Be aware of the deep connection between you. Realize that you chose each other, that you are the best mother for the soul that is taking birth through you. Talk out loud or internally to your child and speak from your deepest heart and soul. Bless your child, yourself, your partner, your family. Thank him or her for coming to be with you. Allow the communion to continue as long as is natural, maybe 10 minutes or more.

When you are ready, slowly return your focus to your breath and the room and open your eyes. Know that you remain connected even in your busiest moments.

NEW MOTHER & BABY

It is truly remarkable how adaptable a woman's body is and how much it changes in one brief year of pregnancy, birth, and lactation. I distinctly recall the day I arrived home with my 3-day-old son, looked in the mirror, and laughed in the delightful realization of what an amazing and wondrous thing a woman's body is. Common sense tells a woman that she has to take it slow and easy when it comes to exercise after her baby is born. She may wish to look and feel as she did before her pregnancy, but the reality is that it took 9 months to make the baby and it will probably take at least that long for her body to return to a prepregnancy state of health and fitness.

Barring complications, most women may begin with pelvic floor exercises (p.25) and gentle exercise within weeks of birth. Women's concerns about exercise in the postnatal phase usually have to do with three basic practicalities: having time for exercise, having the energy, and knowing which exercises will be safe and effective.

Having energy can be a real challenge for a new mother. There is so much to adjust to that it can easily become over-whelming. Suddenly there is a small being who is completely dependent on you. That alone would be enough, but huge hormonal changes are going on in your body that can wreak havoc on your emotional state of mind. You may alternate between feelings of blissful contentment and frenzied anxiety, and everything in between. Just remember, you are handling a lot of change; go easy on yourself and ground yourself in your meditative mind as often as possible.

As for finding time to exercise, find a few minutes here and there for stretching, maybe while waiting for the coffee to brew with your baby safely in a carrier on the kitchen table. Hold onto the table and stretch your lower back (see Preparing for Birth, p.181). In fact, most of these exercises are great for postpartum, with one important difference: the emphasis during pregnancy is on poses and exercises that open the pelvis, such as squats and Butterfly pose; the focus in postpartum is on healing and strengthening the pelvic area and pulling it back together. The postpartum phase is a recovery period. Be gentle with yourself and have patience and appreciation for your body.

Breastfeeding

Hopefully you are breastfeeding your baby; there is nothing like breastfeeding to bond mother and baby. Mother's milk naturally has everything that the baby needs—and the milk is always available! To stay healthy while breastfeeding, remember these two very simple but important points:

• **Eat well.** Eat fruit, vegetables, whole grains, and foods high in protein. Organic milk products, soy products, beans, legumes, nuts, and seeds are your healthiest choices for protein.

• **Rest well.** Rest whenever your baby does, at least for the first few months. Relaxation is important, too. Let your partner have special time with the baby while you take a break and have a warm bath, read, visit a friend, or have a little time to yourself in whatever way you most enjoy.

Special nursing drink

6 oz (180 g) organic milk (dairy or nondairy)
6–8 blanched almonds (soaked and peeled)
2 tsp ghee (purified butter)
1–2 tsp honey
Blend well. Drink this to help produce rich, nourishing milk for your baby. Makes 1 cup.

POSTPARTUM YOGA

If your labor and delivery were uncomplicated, you may be able to exercise within the first few weeks of delivery. Every woman's body and every birthing story is different, so check first with your physician. Go slowly and stay aware of your body as you practice. Stay in a pose for 3–4 breaths to begin with, working up slowly to 15 breaths.

The Kegel exercise is a short, upward vaginal squeeze and release technique. Try to do 100 a day—anytime, anywhere—to regain essential muscle tone after pregnancy.

HAND GRASP

This adjusts the vertebrae of the middle and upper spine, opens the chest and shoulder areas, and counteracts any tendency to slump while breast-feeding or carrying your baby. It may be helpful to use a prop.

Using props
Make your belt short enough so that you can really stretch deeply.

(1) Sit on a chair or on the ground, or stand. Keep your spine straight and chest lifted the entire time to perform this pose. Bend your left elbow and reach your left arm behind your back. Draw the upper part of your arm close to the side of your body. Raise your right arm up.

(2) Bend your right arm at the elbow so that your right hand reaches toward your shoulder blade and faces your back. Interlock your fingers. If they do not reach, touch your fingers together or use a belt or rope (inset). Breathe deeply with your eyes closed for 5–8 breaths, then reverse the hands.

LOCUST LIFTS

Recovering muscle tone after pregnancy is key, especially in the core muscles that support the pelvis and torso. Locust Lifts are particularly beneficial for strengthening and toning the abdominal and back muscles. To build strength and prepare for holding this pose, try inhaling up into the pose and exhaling down several times beforehand.

1. Lie on your front with your arms by your sides, palms facing upward. Rest your chin on the ground.

2. Inhale and simultaneously lift your right leg and your left arm up. Arch your chest and pelvis as you extend up. Inhale and exhale deeply and hold for 5–8 breaths. Then relax down briefly and repeat with the left leg and right arm. Continue for 6–10 breaths.

3. To end, turn your head to one side, place your arms by your sides, and relax.

SPINAL TWIST

This gives a lateral stretch to the vertebrae, back muscles, and hips; keeps the spine elastic; and helps to retain side-to-side mobility. It also massages the abdominal muscles, aids in digestion, and calms nerves.

Date milk

Soothing and delicious, this milk with origins in Ayurveda help babies wean from breastfeeding. It gives energy, provides nourishment, and helps ward off colds.

Heat together: 1 cup (250 ml) organic milk (dairy or nondairy) and 6 dates, sliced in half Simmer on low heat for 20 minutes. Add a little water if needed. Strain. Makes 1 cup.

(1) Sit in Easy pose (p.19) with your spine straight. Raise the right knee. Place the right foot flat on the ground.

(2) Place the right foot on the ground outside your left thigh, your right knee bent over your left leg. Place the right hand on the ground just behind your back. It should bear no weight. Raise the left arm up.

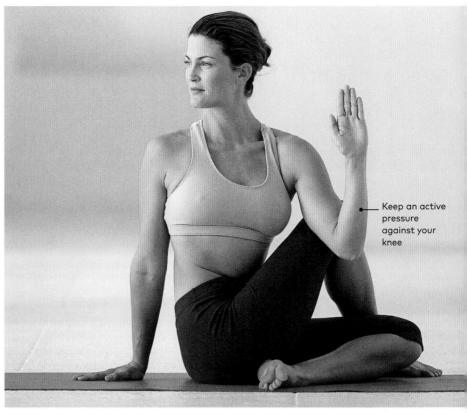

Keep an active pressure against your knee

(3) Bring your left arm over to your right knee. Your left arm will push against your right knee. Your head is erect and turned to look over your right shoulder. Your chest is lifted and the shoulders are parallel to the ground. Hold for 5–10 deep breaths. Release and repeat on the other side.

BUTTERFLY-COCOON

This gentle movement strengthens your navel chakra and abdominal muscles. If your abdominals need more gradual strengthening, straighten your legs to a 90° angle instead, then bring them back into your chest.

(1) Lie on your back and tuck your knees to your chest. Place your hands on your shins, holding your knees in Cocoon pose. Exhale.

Keep the toes pointed

Use the abdominal muscles to control the gradual extension of the legs

(2) Inhale and open your arms out straight to the sides, almost touching the ground. Simultaneously extend your legs straight out to about a 60° angle from the ground into Butterfly pose. On the exhalation, slowly return to Cocoon. Continue for 1–3 minutes.

BABY YOGA

You will have your baby by your side most of the time, so why not enjoy your time together in a way that benefits both of you? When assisting your baby to move her body, never move her with force. Don't be discouraged if she resists: she is adjusting to the wide open spaces of a new life. Help her relax and uncurl and learn about her environment in a natural, flowing way with gentle touch, eye contact, your voice, and your love.

Through the years of mothering and teaching children, this quote from Yogi Bhajan has given me guidance: "Children are super-sensitive, full-fledge people, with high potency antennae that record every vibration within their vicinity, completely and deeply."

HEART CROSSES

Crossing the midline of the body strengthens crossover connections between the right and left brains. This exercise stretches and strengthens your baby's arms and upper back.

① Lay your baby on a blanket facing you and sit or kneel in front of her. Hold her hands and cross her arms over her chest.

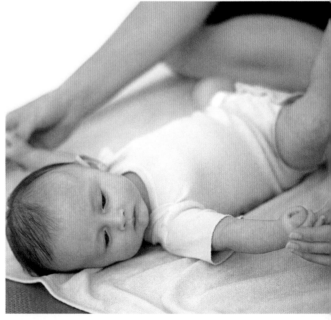

② Bring her arms out to the sides. Chant a mantra such as Sat Nam in rhythm with the movement. Repeat steps 1 and 2 for as long as you both like.

BICYCLES

Moving your baby's legs in a bicycling motion and rocking her knees up to her chest helps to relieve trapped gas. It also helps your baby to strengthen her leg and abdominal muscles.

① Lay your baby on a soft blanket. Smile and look into her eyes. Talk to her about what you are going to do. Gently rotate her legs alternately in a bicycling motion. Sing or chant in rhythm with the motion.

② To end, bring both of her knees up toward her chest and rock her slightly back, so her bottom comes off the floor. Do this a few times, then let her legs relax down.

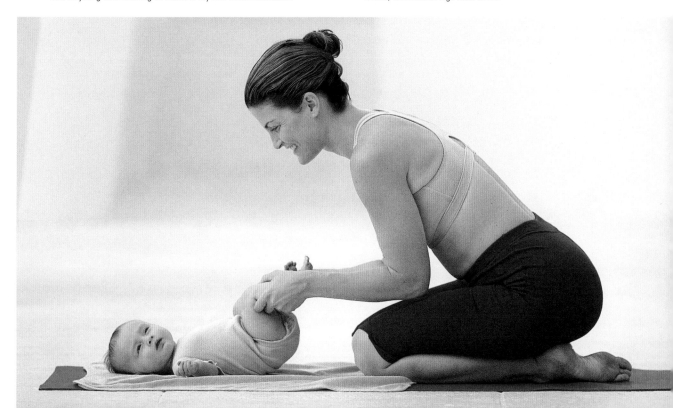

BABY AND ME PELVIC LIFTS

Pelvic Tilts enhance the flexibility in your spine and tone your abdominal and leg muscles. After giving birth, practice Pelvic Tilts against the wall before trying them with your baby.

① Lie on your back with your knees bent and your pelvis tucked forward slightly. Place your baby on your abdomen, facing you and resting against your bent legs. Hold your baby on her shoulders, or if your baby's neck is stable, hold onto her arms.

② Inhale and lift your pelvis slightly, then exhale and bring it back down. Hold your baby steady the entire time. Smile, laugh, and keep eye contact with her. Continue for as long as you both like.

BUNDLE WRAP

In many indigenous cultures, mothers wrap their babies in cloth, with their arms and legs straight down at their sides. This is also a yogic technique that provides cozy security for a baby from 1 or 2 months onward. Cut a piece of lightweight cloth (sheeting works well) in a rectangle long enough to wrap around a few times from shoulder to foot. Lie your baby near one edge with enough cloth to bring across the front side and tuck it between her arm and side. Then roll her up. For a peaceful sleep, hold your baby at your chest, heart to heart, and pat her as you sing or hum. Any resistance she gives to the wrap is beneficial, as it builds muscle and nerve strength. A wrap may be used before nighttime sleep, but your baby should be unwrapped after an hour or so.

THE GRACE OF GOD MEDITATION

This is perfect for a busy new mom. It is quick and potent, and you can do it lying down. It helps to positively channel your emotions. There are two parts, and although it is recommended to do them together, they can be done separately or whenever you have a spare 5 minutes. Remind yourself of your authentic essence as you use the affirmation, "I am the Grace of God." The optimum times for this meditation are at sunrise and sunset, preferably practiced twice a day.

1 Lie on your back with your arms at your sides. Relax your face and body. Take a few deep breaths. Inhale, hold the breath in, and repeat silently to yourself "I am the Grace of God." Exhale and repeat the affirmation silently 10 times. Continue for five breaths. This will make a total 100 times that the mantra/affirmation is repeated.

2 After the cycle is completed, or at a different time of the day, sit in Easy pose. Bring your right hand into Gyan Mudra (p.21). Hold the left hand up by the left shoulder, palm flat and facing forward, as though taking an oath. The chest is lifted and the spine is straight. Your breath is relaxed and normal. Begin with the index finger of the left hand. Tense the finger and repeat out loud, "I am the Grace of God" five times. Do the same with each finger and thumb. Inhale to end and feel the reality of the affirmation you have just repeated. Exhale and relax.

MATURING GRACEFULLY

Many women say that as they grow older, life takes on a richness previously undreamed of—that the second half of life really can be better than the first. Major changes in responsibilities such as children growing up, a secure home, and reevaluating work open the door to new opportunities for women at this stage. How well a woman can appreciate and enjoy the second half of life depends very much on the quality of her health and well-being. This is where yoga plays a part in helping women mature with grace. In this last section, you can practice yoga that helps you maintain strong physical health; glowing inner and outer beauty; and a mind that's clear, calm, and able to live in a timeless state of consciousness.

AGELESS BEAUTY

Staying young for a long time is a wonderful, blessed way to live. As women, we have so much to give as we mature, so much wisdom born of hard-earned experience and loving kindness to share. So let's keep our good health and vitality and reap the profit of a life well-lived. The practices in this part of the book focus on just that. Yoga keeps us well-oiled as we age, and you'll find a few exercises that help prevent arthritis, as well as yoga sequences that help maintain good bone density and help prevent osteoporosis. Just for the fun of it, and because we women love to look and feel beautiful, I've included yoga for your face and a special yoga set for radiant beauty. Enjoy—and feel like the beautiful soul that you are!

BENDING CIRCLES

This exercise aids in the prevention of arthritis. It improves spinal flexibility and helps you feel young and energetic. If you have arthritis or bursitis in your shoulders or back, use slower, smaller movements.

(1) Stand with your feet shoulder-width apart, your spine straight, and your knees soft. Bring your arms straight out to the sides of your body.

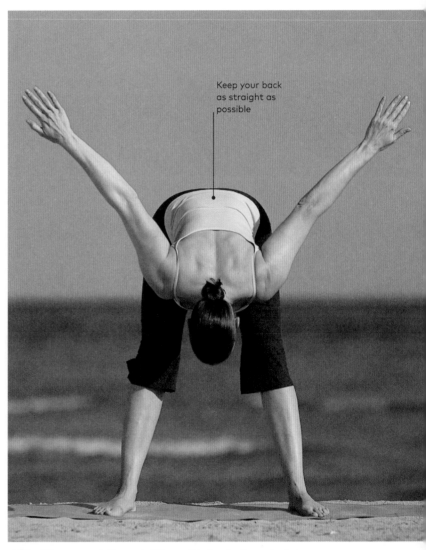

Keep your back as straight as possible

(2) Counting out loud from 1 to 8, begin to bend forward slowly from the waist while moving the arms in forward circles, making the circles about the size of a dinner plate.

(3) When you reach the count of 8, you will be bending forward as far as possible. Then make backward circles with the arms as you slowly rise up again, counting from 8 to 1. Continue for 1–3 minutes.

LIONESS POSE

This pose works on firming your neck muscles, exercises your eye muscles, and opens your throat. The strong breathing that you practice in this exercise releases toxins from the body.

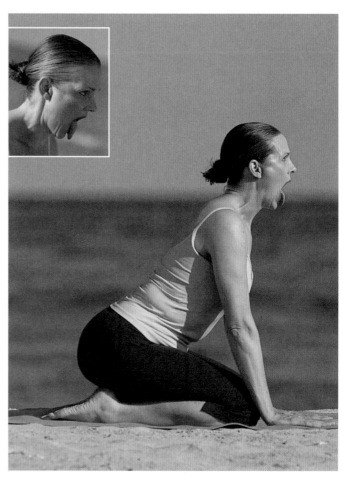

① Sit on your knees in Rock pose (p.20), your hands resting on your thighs. Then place your hands on the ground in front of your knees, palms down.

② Draw your chin in toward your chest. Stretch out your tongue as far as possible (inset). Open your eyes wide and breathe through your mouth. Roar like a lioness. Continue for 1 minute.

QUEEN DANCER

Originally called King Dancer, Queen Dancer is a more appropriate name for this women's yoga book! It gives you a sense of elation and power, rejuvenates your spine and internal organs, and improves your sense of balance. A good sense of balance can help prevent falls, which can be a serious problem as we age, especially if bone density is weakened.

What is the relationship between yoga and healthy bone density? Bone production is stimulated when tension and resistance are applied on the tendons that attach to bones. Yoga, being weight-bearing, does just that.

① Stand straight with your arms at your sides. If you are a beginner, use a wall in front of you as a support for balance.

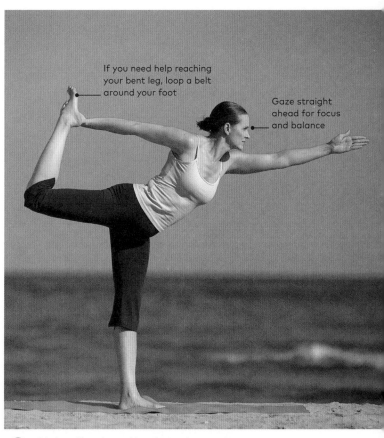

If you need help reaching your bent leg, loop a belt around your foot

Gaze straight ahead for focus and balance

② Bend your right knee so that your right foot is behind you. Take hold of the inner side of your foot with your right hand. Straighten your elbow. Stretch your left arm up close to your ear.

③ Inhale and lean forward, lengthening the spine. At the same time, lift your bent leg and arm up behind you as high as possible. Breathe deeply and look straight ahead. Hold for 5–15 breaths. Then repeat the posture on the opposite arm and leg.

PLANK

This pose strengthens the arms and legs and builds upper body muscle mass, which is a factor in helping to increase bone density. Spend a few moments in Child's pose (p.63) afterward to relax the lower spine.

A challenging asana, Plank helps to strengthen and tone muscles in the arms, legs, and upper body, building bone density to reduce the risk of conditions such as osteoporosis.

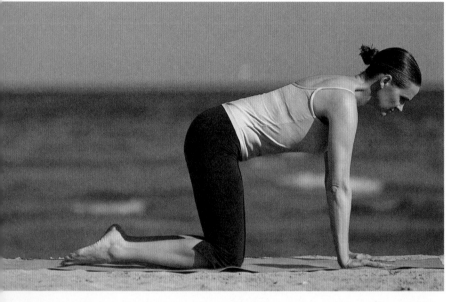

① This pose is best done on a yoga mat. Begin on your hands and knees.

② Extend your right leg back and place your toes only on the ground, then extend the left leg back. Balance your weight on your toes.

Easy-does-it version

Begin on your hands and knees. Lean forward
onto your arms and stretch out your torso so
that your body is in a straight angle from
knees to shoulders. Your shoulders are directly
over your elbows, with your head facing the
ground and your chin tucked in slightly.
Continue to hold for 2–8 deep breaths.

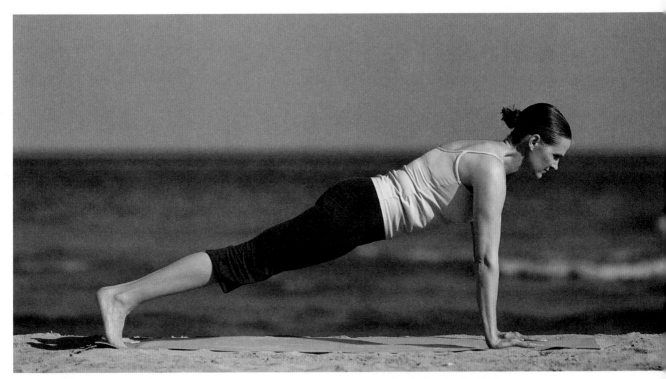

(3) Lift your torso as you straighten your legs. Keep your shoulders directly over your hands. You body forms a straight angle from shoulders to heels. Tuck your chin slightly toward your neck and feel a stretch at the back of the neck. Continue to hold for 2–8 deep breaths. To come out of the pose, relax your knees onto the ground and come back to the starting position.

FOR RADIANT HEALTH

This short set brings vibrant, radiant health and helps develop a meditative mind; it increases your beauty both physically and mentally. To become beautiful inside and out, you need a flow of pranic energy to brighten your eyes and skin and generate glowing health.

1 LION FLEX

This exercise increases flexibility in the spine, which is the true measure of youthfulness. Be aware of flexing each vertebra of your spine in a flowing movement.

① Sit on your heels with a straight spine. Place the palms of your hands on the ground just in front of the knees. Bring your neck vertebrae in line with your spine by lifting your head and tucking the chin in slightly.

② Begin flexing your spine to its maximum capacity, keeping the elbows straight as you flex: inhale and arch your spine, lifting your chest while keeping your head level.

③ Exhale as you round your spine so that your chest curls inward. Keep a constant rhythm as you repeat the pose. You may begin to sweat lightly on the forehead and spine. Continue for 2–3 minutes.

2 VENUS LOCK STRETCH

This exercise brings circulation to your face and cheeks. Try smiling while you breathe in this exercise; the best face lift you can have is to smile as often as possible. Besides, you cannot think a negative thought when you are smiling—try it and see!

① Sit in Rock pose. Bring the hands behind your back in Venus Lock: interlace the fingers so that the right thumb presses into the webbing between the left thumb and left index finger.

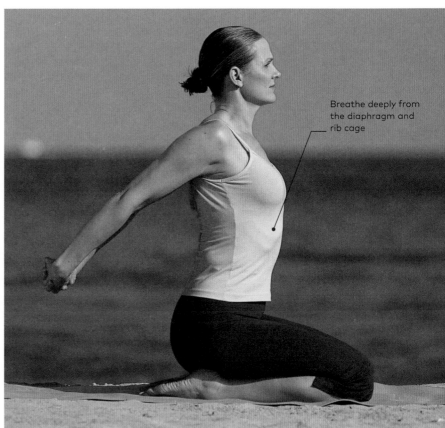

Breathe deeply from the diaphragm and rib cage

② Straighten your arms behind you, lifting as high as you can without straining. The arms are positioned so that the palms are facing your back. Breathe and relax into the position for 1–2 minutes.

③ Relax your arms down and sit restfully in Rock pose for 2 minutes, breathing normally.

3 LIFT AND HOLD

This pose helps to relieve headaches. It also stretches and strengthens the sciatic nerves in the legs. There is a strong, automatic tendency to shake in this position, which strengthens the entire nervous system.

① Sit with a straight spine and your legs outstretched in front of you with your heels together. Your hands are flat on the ground beside your hips.

② Place your hands slightly behind your hips and lean back, keeping your chest lifted. Point your toes.

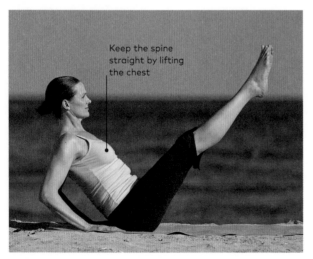

Keep the spine straight by lifting the chest

③ Bending your elbows, lean back as you inhale and raise your legs slowly to a 60° angle and hold. Keep your legs together and breathe deeply for 1–3 minutes.

④ Come out of the pose by relaxing your legs down onto the ground. Relax and sit straight or rest in a Forward Bend for a few seconds.

4 FEET UP

Fifty powerful and continuous repetitions of Breath of Fire while in this position cleanse and improve blood circulation. It cleans the lungs and stimulates the prana so that you are able to retain your youth and power.

(1) Sit with a straight spine and your legs outstretched in front of you with your heels together. Place your hands slightly behind your hips.

(2) Bend your elbows. Lean back with a straight spine. Then bend your knees and bring them as close to your chest as possible. Hold your feet 6 in (15 cm) off the ground and balance. Begin 50 powerful repetitions of Breath of Fire. Inhale deeply, exhale, and relax your legs onto the ground. Rest in a Forward Bend for a few seconds if you wish.

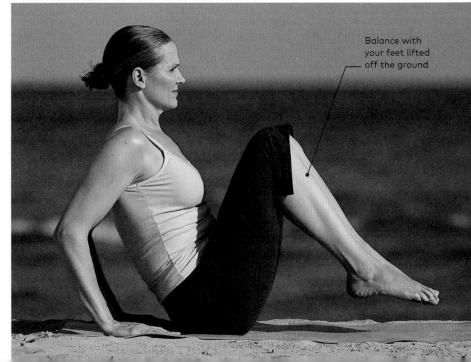

Balance with your feet lifted off the ground

5 FORWARD STRETCH

This exercise invigorates the liver and spleen. Pressing your toes with your fingers stimulates reflexology points that help stimulate brain activity. The top back area of the big toe stimulates the pituitary gland. Chanting cleans the lungs and strongly stimulates the pranic life force so that you can retain your youth, power, and work potency.

As you hold this posture, chant the sound *Hum*. It means "we," and it helps to take you out of your own smallness and feel a unity with all life. The "mmm" sound is continuous.

1. Extend your legs straight in front of you and place your hands on the ground by your hips. Lift up slightly so that your pelvis straightens and you sit on your buttocks.

Lengthen your spine and stretch it up fully

Keep your arms straight

2. Reach up, then bend forward and catch your toes and press them. If you cannot reach your toes, loop a belt around your feet and hold onto it with both hands. Pull your neck back and tuck your chin in toward your neck. With your eyes closed, gently roll the eyes upward, as though looking through the forehead. Breathe for 1–2 minutes and chant Hum.

FOR HAPPINESS, LONGEVITY, AND BEAUTY

This is a beautiful meditation. It is said to have the ability to make a woman feel happy and extend her life. The mudra (hand position) and breath affect the brain chemistry in ways that allow you to feel cozy and relaxed, and your face reflects an innocent charm. This is a relaxing meditation, perfect to do before bedtime or to help you feel refreshed after work. Do not practice it if you have work to do. You may like to practice for 11 minutes, a complete meditation cycle of time.

1 Sit comfortably in a meditative pose with your spine straight. Bring your hands in front of you so that the palms of the hands face each other. Curl the fingers of your left hand into a fist, then wrap the fingers of your right hand around the left with the heels of the hands touching. When you look down at your hands, your left index finger should be closest to you. Bring your thumbs together so the sides are touching, then rest them on the index finger of the left hand. They should not touch the right index finger at all. An air space is naturally created between the hands.

2 With the hands positioned 8–10 in (21–24 cm) from the face at mouth level, begin inhaling deeply through the nose and exhaling through the mouth, directing the air through the opening created between your thumbs. Exhale completely. Close your eyes and continue the breath meditation for however long you wish—even until you fall asleep.

Wrap the fingers of the right hand around the left

The thumbs rest on the left index finger

LIVING IN THE MOMENT

Right now is the only time you actually exist. The past exists only in memory, and the future only in your mind's projection. Being "present" to the present is truly living. What does it feel like to be present? Some describe it as feeling grounded, stable, expansive, and peaceful, deeply peaceful. There is no need for judgment, guilt, anger—or even patience—fortitude, and forgiveness, as they all stem from resistance to what "is." Being present is being with life as it is and allowing it simply because it is what it is! In being present to the eternal Now, you experience what in yoga is called Shunia, the zero point, where the neutral mind, the loving heart, and the expanded awareness exist as one.

THE WARRIOR SEQUENCE

The dance of breath, movement, and awareness is the signature of a vinyasa. In this powerful vinyasa, be mindful of the interplay of breath and movement. Pause the breath at the end of both the inhalation and exhalation. In that pause of 1 or 2 seconds, relate to the stillness inside, outside, and all around.

Practice Full Warrior for a week or so, then add Extended Warrior, and so on, until you know the entire sequence.

1 FULL WARRIOR

The vertebrae of the midspine are flexed and digestion is stimulated in this pose. Energy is also circulated throughout the middle and upper back.

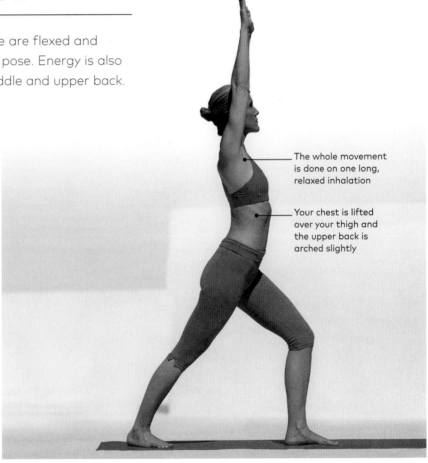

The whole movement is done on one long, relaxed inhalation

Your chest is lifted over your thigh and the upper back is arched slightly

① Stand with your left leg 2–4 ft (60–120 cm) forward and your right foot behind you, turned out slightly. Your arms are by your sides. Your back leg is the grounding element in this pose: keep your right leg strong and maintain a lifting feeling in the left knee.

② On a slow, deep inhalation, bend the left knee so that it is directly above your ankle. Lift your arms up close to your ears, palms facing forward. As the movement and breath end, tilt the chin up slightly and focus on the horizon. Exhale and return to the starting position. Repeat 2–3 times, then change legs and repeat.

2 EXTENDED WARRIOR

This pose strengthens the spine and legs and tones the abdominal muscles and nervous system. Keep the mind focused and the eyes gazing forward as you practice Extended Warrior.

Practice this sequence 2–3 times, then rest in the counterpose (p.220) before repeating the sequence again with the right foot in front.

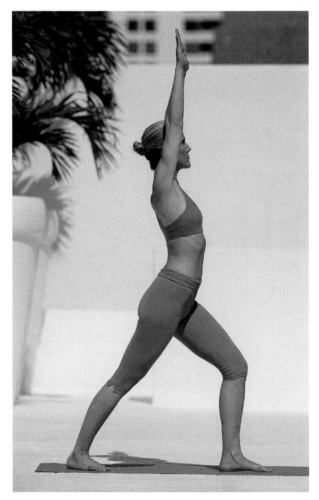

① Stand with your left leg 2–4 ft (60–120 cm) forward and your right foot behind you, turned out slightly. Your arms are by your sides.

② Inhale and come up into Full Warrior pose: bend the left knee so that it is directly above your ankle and lift your arms up close to your ears, palms facing forward.

Your body forms a straight angle from the spine through the arms and hands

Maintain a stable base and lift the muscles around the knees

(4) Inhale deeply and return to Full Warrior position as before.

(5) Exhale and bring the arms down, returning to the starting position.

(3) Exhale and come into Extended Warrior: maintain a stable base with your legs while reaching your arms forward at a 60° angle. Your chest comes out over your thigh, arms still hugging the ears, and the spine and neck are aligned.

3 WARRIOR BEND

This pose invigorates and refreshes the mind since it increases the blood supply to the brain, greatly enhancing concentration and mental capacity. Adding this forward bend into the Warrior sequence stretches and strengthens the lower and upper spine. If you have a weak back, bring your arms down toward the ground before you bend fully forward. Rise up slowly if you begin to feel dizzy or off-balance.

Continue to practice all eight steps of Warrior Bend 2–3 times with the left foot in front, then rest in the counterpose (p.220) for 30 seconds to 1 minute. Repeat the sequence with the right foot in front.

① Stand with your left leg 2–4 ft (60–120 cm) forward and your right foot behind you, turned out slightly. Your arms are by your sides.

② Inhale and come up into Full Warrior pose: bend the left knee so that it is directly above your ankle, and lift your arms up close to your ears, palms facing forward.

③ Exhale into Extended Warrior: reach your arms and upper body forward so that your chest is over your thigh, your arms are by your ears, and the spine and neck are aligned.

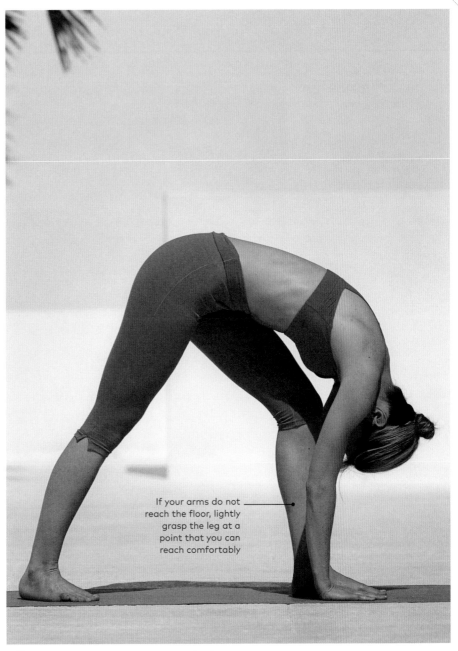

If your arms do not reach the floor, lightly grasp the leg at a point that you can reach comfortably

(4) Inhale and return to Full Warrior position.

(5) Exhale, and with your upper arms still close by your ears, bend forward in Head-to-Knee position. Reach your arms to the ground and rest them there. Continue to ground yourself firmly through the back leg.

▶

Inhale and return to Full Warrior position as before.

(7) Exhale and return to Extended Warrior pose, maintaining a stable base with your legs while reaching your arms and upper body forward.

(8) Inhale and return to Full Warrior position. Exhale and return to the starting position. Repeat 2–3 times.

NADABRAHMA MEDITATION

Through this meditation, you learn to listen—
to yourself, your partner, and everyone you meet.
Ultimately you learn to listen to, and be guided
by, the soundless sound of the universe.

1 Sit in a relaxed position with your eyes closed
and lips together, relaxed. Start humming loudly
enough to be heard by others and to create a
vibration throughout your body. Visualize a hollow
tube or empty vessel, filled only with the vibrations
of the humming. A point will come when the
humming continues by itself and you become the
listener. There is no special breathing. Alter the
pitch or move your body smoothly and slowly
if you feel it. Continue for 30 minutes.

2 The second stage of the meditation is divided
into two 7½-minute sections. For the first half,
move the hands, palms up, in an outward circular
motion. Starting at the navel, both hands
move forward, then divide to make two large
circles mirroring each other on the left and
right. The movement should be so slow that at
times there will appear to be no movement
at all. Feel that you are giving energy outward
to the universe.

3 After 7½ minutes, turn the hands so that the
palms are down and move them in the opposite
direction. Now the hands come together toward
the navel and divide outward to the sides of the
body. Feel that you are taking energy in. As in the
previous movement, move extremely slowly. As in
the first part of the meditation, don't inhibit any
soft, slow movements of the rest of your body with
these hand movements. Sit or lie absolutely quiet
and still for 15 minutes.

Giving motion: circle hands outward, palms up

Receiving motion: circle hands inward, palms down

4 WARRIOR BALANCE

This additional pose may be added to the vinyasa at the intermediate level. For extra balancing support, position yourself near a wall so that when you lean forward, your fingertips touch the wall.

As an alternative, try any and all of the Warrior sequences with the hands extended in Prayer pose.

① Stand with your left leg forward, right foot behind and turned out slightly, and arms by your sides.

② Inhale into Full Warrior pose as before.

③ Exhale into Extended Warrior pose as before, maintaining a stable base with your legs.

④ Inhale into Full Warrior pose as before.

⑤ Exhale and lift the heel of your right foot up and lean forward with the spine lengthened. Keep your arms up and reach out and up as you shift your weight to your left foot and lift your right foot off the ground.

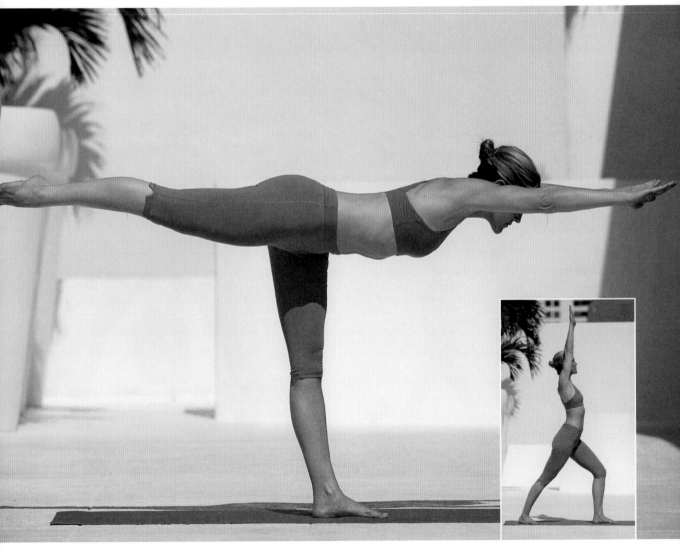

⑥ Lift your back leg so that your body forms a straight line from your hands to your toes. It may help to point the toes of your lifted leg. Gaze ahead as you feel the extension in your torso, arms, and leg.

⑦ Bend your left knee and lower your right leg. Inhale into Full Warrior pose. ▶

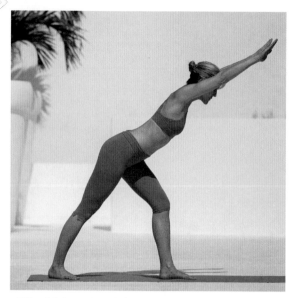

8 Exhale into Extended Warrior pose as before, maintaining a stable base with your legs.

9 Inhale into Full Warrior pose as before.

10 Exhale and come back to the starting position to end. Practice 2–3 rounds, then rest in the counterpose before repeating the sequence with the right leg forward.

5 WARRIOR COUNTERPOSE

This allows your body to stretch and relax in the opposite direction from the Warrior sequence. Practice it after each round or at the end of the set.

With your legs straddled, pivot your feet so they are parallel to each other. Bend forward and rest your hands on the floor, or just allow your arms to hang down. Relax in the forward bending position, yield to gravity, and let all tension go. Smile from the inside! Relax for 30 seconds to 2 minutes.

MOMENT-TO-MOMENT PRACTICE OF PEACE

This practice draws upon elements of present moment awareness and mindfulness. If you wish, you can record this meditation in your own voice and then play it back to practice. To deepen the effect, pauses have been added to allow the previous practice to subtly resonate in your awareness. Stay with the sensation until you feel it settle into a deep stillness, then move on to the next part.

Observing and Allowing

Focus your awareness on your sensations. The feelings in your physical body, your breath, the sounds. Allow them all equally, without any special focus on any one of them. Let thoughts arise and watch them, as waves washing up on the shore of your awareness (pause).

Some feelings and thoughts that arise may be painful. Experiment with allowing the pain to be. Everything is allowed; nothing is judged. See that it cannot hurt you to let it be (pause).

After a few moments of observing and allowing the pain, a new element of acceptance is introduced and pain with total acceptance is no longer pain (pause).

Being in the Empty Space of Creation

Settle into your inner self. Experience a feeling of extending out in all directions. In observing these sensations, experience a deep space around you and inside you—a profound stillness and silence.

Let a few seconds go by and realize that the "I" that seems to be you did not exist for a time. There is only beingness in this space. Experience this expanded awareness as an emptiness in which all potential of creation exists. Know that anything is possible in this creative emptiness and that it exists all the time, whether you experience it or not (pause).

Adding Intention to Your Awareness

Without effort, allow intention into the empty space of all possibilities. The intention may feel like a bubble rising from the water's depth to break on the surface. Insights that are related to the intention may come forward into your consciousness. You may have a sense of what would heal a particular situation or person or an insight into how to move forward in your life. Remain neutral and nonresistant as intention and insight stabilize in your awareness (pause).

Living Life with Awareness

After a sitting practice, hold the intention of moving through your life with awareness of each moment. Bit by bit, find your way to the practice of peace until it becomes a way of life.

INDEX

About the author

Shakta Khalsa has been practicing and teaching yoga since 1976, specializing in women's yoga and yoga for children. She is a professional yoga teacher at the highest level (E-RYT-500) and the author of best-selling yoga books, including *Kundalini Yoga* (DK) and *The Yoga Way to Radiance* (Llewellyn Publications). She is also the founder and director of Radiant Child Yoga, a distinguished teacher-training program for working with children, teens, and families. Shakta was named in the top five kundalini teachers in *Yoga Journal*'s who's who.

Resources
Music
Women's Yoga Music, a full-length album compiled by Shakta Khalsa and the perfect companion to *Yoga for Women*. Available as a CD or MP3. To order, go to www.spiritvoyage.com or www.childrensyoga.com

Websites
www.childrensyoga.com
Information about Radiant Child Yoga, the author's Yoga Alliance-certified school and training program, including free resources for teaching babies through teens, and an online shop with digital music, videos, and books.

www.shaktawrites.com
The author's uplifting journey into becoming more of her authentic self, as expressed through poetry and prose.

Acknowledgments
Author's acknowledgments
I am deeply grateful for the love and support of my teacher, Yogi Bhajan; my husband, Kartar Singh Khalsa; and my son, Ram Das Singh Khalsa. My gratitude goes to the wonderful women whose insight, creativity, and plain hard work shaped this book: Gillian Roberts, Mary-Clare Jerram, Susannah Steel, Claire Legemah, Karen Sawyer, and LaVonne Carlson; to the talented photographer, Russell Sadur, and his assistant, Nina Duncan; to Cindy Andrews for hair and makeup; and to the superb models who gave their best to this book. My thanks to all who offered their expertise: Patricia Miller, Kay Hawkins, Dr. Nirmala Lamaye, Bonnie Berk, and Gururam Kaur. Special thanks go to Satya Kaur Khalsa for making KRI a joy to work with.

Dedicated with love and gratitude to Yogi Bhajan, my spiritual teacher and master of kundalini yoga, and to my mother, Grace Meyers, for her unfailing love and support.

Publisher's acknowledgments
Thanks to Dawn Young and Anna Benjamin for design assistance, and Hilary Bird for the index.
All photographs © Dorling Kindersley, except the photograph of the author on p.6, Gurusurya Photography. For further information visit www.dkimages.com
Photography: photographer Russell Sadur, assisted by Nina Duncan; photographic production and location services in Miami, Sharon Weems.
Models: Clinton Archambault, Gurmeet K. Cheng, Rudy Estripeant, Mia Rosen Glick (Fateh Kaur), Sarah Ruby Glick, Catherine Goodrum, Anna Karina Gutierrez, Anastasia Levinson (Siri Adi Kaur), Mary E. Schroeder, Spencer Singer, Kelly Smith-Beany, Cate Williams
Hair and makeup: Cindy Andrews
Stylist: Liz Hancock
Yoga mats kindly supplied by: Hugger Mugger Yoga Products www.huggermugger.com
Yoga props kindly supplied by: Yoga Matters www.yogamatters.co.uk
Leisure clothing kindly supplied by: Toast www.toa.st/uk
Nadabrahama Meditation (p.217) reprinted with permission by Osho International (www.osho.com).
Pranayama to Expel Negativity and Disease (p.163) reprinted with permission from *A Year with the Master* by Atma Singh and Guruprem Kaur Khalsa

SECOND EDITION
Senior Editor Dawn Titmus
Senior Designer Glenda Fisher
Editor Claire Cross
US Editor Kayla Dugger
Designer Mandy Earey
Pre-Production Producer Heather Blagden
Producer Rebecca Parton
Jacket Designer Nicola Powling
Jacket Coordinator Lucy Philpott
Managing Editor Stephanie Farrow
Managing Art Editor Christine Keilty
Art Director Maxine Pedliham
Publishing Director Mary-Clare Jerram

DK INDIA
Pre-Production Manager Sunil Sharma
Senior DTP Designer Pushpak Tyagi
DTP Designers Manish Upreti, Rajdeep Singh, Anurag Trivedi, Satish Gaur

This American Edition, 2019
First American Edition, 2002
Published in the United States by DK Publishing
1450 Broadway, Suite 801, New York, NY 10018

A catalog record for this book
is available from the Library of Congress.
ISBN 978-1-4654-9167-1

Printed and bound in China

A WORLD OF IDEAS:
SEE ALL THERE IS TO KNOW

www.dk.com